You Are Never Alone: Prayers and Meditations to Sustain You Through Breast Cancer

By
Maureen Murray

Oncology Nursing Society
Pittsburgh, PA

ONS Publishing Division
Publisher: Leonard Mafrica, MBA, CAE
Director, Commercial Publishing: Barbara Sigler, RN, MNEd
Production Manager: Lisa M. George
Staff Editor: Lori Wilson
Creative Services Assistant: Dany Sjoen

You Are Never Alone: Prayers and Meditations to Sustain You Through Breast Cancer

Library of Congress Control Number: 2003109687

ISBN 1-890504-40-8

Publisher's Note

This book is published by the Oncology Nursing Society (ONS). ONS neither represents nor guarantees that the practices described herein will, if followed, ensure safe and effective patient care. The recommendations contained in this book reflect ONS's judgment regarding the state of general knowledge and practice in the field as of the date of publication. The recommendations may not be appropriate for use in all circumstances. Those who use this book should make their own determinations regarding specific safe and appropriate patient-care practices, taking into account the personnel, equipment, and practices available at the hospital or other facility at which they are located. The author and publisher cannot be held responsible for any liability incurred as a consequence from the use or application of any of the contents of this book. Figures and tables are used as examples only. They are not meant to be all-inclusive, nor do they represent endorsement of any particular institution by ONS. Mention of specific products and opinions related to those products do not indicate or imply endorsement by ONS.

ONS publications are originally published in English. The ONS Board of Directors has granted permission for foreign translation. (Individual tables and figures that are reprinted or adapted require additional permission from the original source.) However, because translations from English may not always be accurate and precise, ONS disclaims any responsibility for inaccurate translations. Readers relying on precise information should check the original English version.

Printed in the United States of America

Oncology Nursing Society
Integrity • Innovation • Stewardship • Advocacy • Excellence • Inclusiveness

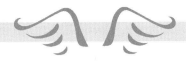

Table of Contents

Preface ix

Acknowledgments xv

Introduction to Prayers 1

Part One: A Journey You Did Not
Choose to Take 3

This section includes the early part of the journey from the shock of hearing a cancer diagnosis, to the search for an excellent surgeon, to the difficult task of telling your children.

While Waiting for Pathology Results 4
When the Diagnosis Is Breast Cancer 6
For Strength to See Beyond Fear 8
Before Telling Your Partner 10
Before Telling Your Children 12
To Find the Right Surgeon 16
While in the Waiting Room 18
To Keep the Statistics in Perspective 20
For the Wisdom to Make Correct
    Medical Choices 22
When You Are a Single Mother 24
When You Are a Young Single Woman
    With Breast Cancer 26
For Grandmothers With Breast Cancer 28

Part Two: Gathering Your Strength for Traveling Through Uncertain Times 31

This section includes the middle part of the journey from the time immediately before surgery through waiting for pathology results.

For Your Surgeon 32
For Concerns About Anesthesia 34
The Night Before Surgery 36
Before Leaving for the Hospital
    for Surgery 38
In the Surgical Holding Area 40
To Be Said With Your Surgeon 42
To Be Said for You While You Are
    in Surgery 44
For Your Nurses 46
Thanksgiving After Surgery 48
If You Learn That You Need
    Chemotherapy 50

Part Three: Continuing Your Pilgrimage Toward Wholeness and Healing 53

This section includes the petitions for the later stage of the journey, such as dealing with various treatments, managing fatigue and discouragement, and hanging on even though it feels like its lasting forever.

To Accept the Changes in Your Body 54
Before Seeing Your Oncologist 56
Before Radiation Treatment 58
Before a Chemotherapy Session 60
For the Strength to Get Through
    the Day 62
When It Is Difficult to Eat 64

When You Must Take Ongoing
　Medication 66
When Your Children Are Sad and
　Concerned About You 68
When You Are in Pain 70
When Treatment Seems Never Ending 72
For Strength for Loved Ones 74
For Your Support Group 76

Part Four: The Road Ahead 79

This section covers the time when treatment is over, life appears to resume a normal course, and the survivor continues to reflect on the experience and consider the impact on her life.

To Accept That Things Are Different 80
Survivor's Prayer of Thanksgiving 82
For the Courage to Change Your Life 84
Prayer Before a Mammogram 86
When You Have a Recurrence 88

Part Five: For Any Time You Need Encouragement 91

This large section includes prayers that are appropriate for any stage of the journey, and they may be interspersed as needed throughout the other sections.

For Long, Dark Evenings 92
In the Middle of the Night (or When You
　Cannot Sleep) 94
For the Strength to Put It Out of Your
　Mind for a While 96
To Get Through the Holidays (and Other
　Special Occasions) 98

When You Are Overwhelmed 100

When You Are Medically Fine but
Still Worried 102

When You Are Struggling to Accept
Help Graciously 104

When You Are Tired of Talking About It 106

When You Are Down 108

When You Are Angry 110

When You Need Mental Clarity 112

When Important Relationships
Are Strained 114

For the Strength to Take Good Care
of Yourself 116

For the Return of a Sense of Humor 118

When God Seems Far Away 120

When You Feel Like Crying 122

For a Friend Who Is Newly Diagnosed 124

For All Women With Breast Cancer 126

For the Wisdom to Find the Good in
This Experience 128

Thanksgiving for Supportive Family 130

Thanksgiving for Supportive Friends 132

Thanksgiving for Faithful Pets 134

Thanksgiving for Everyday Joys 136

Introduction to Meditations 139

**Part Six: Meditations to Calm
Your Spirit 141**

*These meditations are designed to supplement the prayers.
There is a suggestion at the end of each prayer directing
the reader to a meditation that will carry forward the intent of the prayer.*

Place Your Cares on the Altar of God 142

Direct Treatments to Their Target 143

Create a Veil of Love for Your Head 145

Connecting With Your Angel 146

Cloak Yourself With Courage 147

Seeking Peace of Mind and Heart 149

Wrap Your Children in a Quilt
    of God's Love 150

Remember the Gift of Laughter 151

Seeking Solid Ground 153

Remember the Gift of Joy 154

Sing a Song of Thanksgiving 155

Transform Resentment Into Resolve 157

Activate Your Healing Energy 158

Feel the Hand of God Upon Your Face 159

Call Forth Light in the Midst of Darkness ... 161

Seeing the Big Picture 162

Open Your Heart to Wisdom 163

Search for Sun in Gray Skies 165

Glorify All of God's Creatures 166

Surround Caregivers With Grace 167

Staying on Course 169

Bearing a Message of God's Love 170

Part Seven: Prayer Resources to Ensure That You Are Never Alone 173

There are several hundred religious communities in the United States and around the world that offer perpetual, around-the-clock prayer. Following is a sampling of groups who pray for all women who have breast cancer. You are indeed never alone.

Guidelines for Prayer Resources 175

Prayer Resources 178

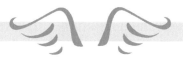

Preface

This project evolved from a personal journey that I never intended to take—the diagnosis and treatment of breast cancer. I offer it as a traveling companion for all women who walk that challenging path. My hope is that it will serve as an accessible friend and personal support group for the more than two million women who live with breast cancer, including the additional 260,000 who were diagnosed in 2003. Its conversational prayers and meditations for specific situations—from diagnosis to surgery to aftermath—and its information about religious communities that pray for women with breast cancer provide a haven of security and comfort.

You Are Never Alone is a constant companion for the patient with breast cancer—in the middle of the night, in the midst of treatment, midway through a busy day—any time the reality of her situation floods her being with uncertainty and fear. The colloquial nature of the prayers that are included stems from my profound belief in a personal God who hears prayer and who maintains a constant presence in our lives.

After my diagnosis of breast cancer, I realized that the most difficult part of the journey was the feeling of traveling down an unfamiliar and frightening road alone. My spouse's support was unwavering, my children and friends rose above and beyond, but there were still times when I was overcome with dread, especially at night during those stark hours that challenge the clock. I searched for uplifting reading material to ease my anxiety. I wanted to pray, but sometimes struggled to find the right words or the written prayers for my specific situation. I longed for simple meditations to focus my energy on healing. Ultimately, I felt called to create a resource that would address those needs and fulfill them with compassion, candor, and simplicity. I hope that I have achieved that goal.

These prayers and guided images were written in a style that is comfortable for me. If the wording feels cumbersome or uncomfortable in any way in any prayer, I encourage women who read this book to substitute words that are familiar and feel right to them. Make the prayers your own by tailoring them to your individual needs.

Shortly after my breast cancer diagnosis, a friend created a prayer chain for me. She contacted friends who agreed to pray at specific times of the day and even located a few self-described insomniacs who volunteered to pray during the night. Knowing that I was receiving constant prayer moved me beyond measure. I knew that God was always with me, and the reality of having people praying for me filled me with relief and gratitude. By sharing information about groups who pray unceasingly, *You Are Never Alone* provides readers with deeply comforting knowledge that they are being remembered in prayer at all times of the day and night. They will know, beyond a doubt, that they are never alone.

My head and heart were both attuned to the powerful physical, mental, emotional, and spiritual benefits of prayer. I knew from personal experience that prayer reduced my feelings of powerlessness over situations that were beyond my control. The act of praying—of *doing* something—transforms us from passive to active, from acceptance to engagement. Focus can be contained rather than scattered. Prayer—be it for a decrease in fear or an actual cure—has the ability to channel energy in a concrete way that anchors us when we feel adrift. I found prayer to be an enormous source of comfort.

Prayer also greatly increased my sense of hope. It uplifted and encouraged me during this difficult time. When we say a prayer of petition, we declare our belief in the possibility that our situation will improve. Research studies consistently show that the expectation of a favorable outcome or an optimistic outlook enables people to weather setbacks more effectively. Prayer helped me to cultivate optimism.

People who pray regularly report enhanced feelings of well-being and life satisfaction. They derive deep satisfaction from a focused and intentional connection with the Divine. They are joined to something much bigger than themselves, and this brings an expanded perspective to their lives. When I prayed, I no longer felt isolated, alienated, or alone. Rather, I gained an ongoing sense of the presence of God.

The medical benefits of prayer were important to me, too. I read about some of the research from prestigious medical schools about the positive effects of prayer. A widely publicized study about the effects of intercessory prayer (praying for someone) at San Francisco General Hospital concluded that CCU patients who were prayed for—unbeknownst to them or staff—required less medication and fewer breathing tubes. A Duke University study of 1,700 older people revealed that people who attended weekly church services had lower levels of interleukin-6, a protein linked to age-related disorders.

A 1995 study from Dartmouth College monitored 232 patients after open-heart surgery and concluded that people with deep religious connections and social support had a six-month survival rate that was 12 times higher than those who did not. In a Georgetown University Medical School study, patients with rheumatoid arthritis reported physical, emotional, and spiritual improvement after four days of intercessory prayer. I was especially interested in a study of women with breast cancer that was conducted at the University of Texas Health Science Center at San Antonio. The researchers concluded that "religiousness" contributed to hope, a primary coping tool for cancer. Prayer helped me to feel like I was collaborating in the healing process.

Despite the many benefits of prayer, it does not guarantee a physical cure. That is a sensitive issue. There is a fundamental difference between curing—the elimination of the disease—and healing—a restoration of balance among mind, body, and spirit. Although it is more common to petition God for a cure, we know that does not always happen. There are many cases where symptoms remain, but healing is evident in the form of peace of mind, renewed energy, and increased perspective. I found it important to keep in mind, and to appreciate, that the benefits of prayer can occur at several levels. That awareness motivated me to include a spirit of gratitude in every prayer.

You Are Never Alone is more than a collection of prayers and meditations. It is a heartfelt *mission*. When adverse events slam into our lives, after our initial reaction, we must choose how to use the experience. This book gleans the good from a stressful and frightening process and offers it to other women as a source of encouragement, fellowship, and strength. No woman with breast cancer needs to feel isolated by fear and uncertainty when she can reach for *You Are Never Alone*. She can select relevant and encouraging prayers for her specific circumstances, focus her mind on calming meditations, and consult the resource section if she wishes to connect with religious groups and place prayer requests for herself and/or other women with breast cancer. Each reader should be assured and may take comfort from knowing that I visit these sites on a regular basis and request prayers for all women with breast cancer, so at any given time—day or night—one or more members of these organizations is lifting her up in prayer.

I offer my ongoing and heartfelt prayers for all women whose lives have been affected by breast cancer. May God bless you with abundant comfort, compassion, and healing on each step of your journey.

Maureen Murray

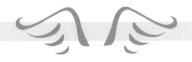

Acknowledgments

Every book that reaches print reflects the efforts of a team of faithful supporters, helpers, and in this case, pray-ers. I am grateful to the following friends, colleagues, and loved ones who helped me to make this project possible.

Kathy Friday, whose prayer chain provided the loving and immeasurable comfort that led to the inspiration for this book. I offer my deepest gratitude to all members of the prayer team.

Colleen McKenna, whose early response to the concept of this book was heartfelt and encouraging. Barbara Sigler, at the Oncology Nursing Society (ONS), whose positive reaction and tremendous work and support kept my motivation high. Lisa George and Lori Wilson, editors at ONS, for their exceptional skills and encouragement. Dany Sjoen, for beautiful and creative design work. Vicki Vogeler, for careful manuscript preparation, excellent editorial support, and reader reaction. Sister Marita Ganley, SC, for encouraging me to write, to go deeper, to serve God, and to live with joy. Dear friends, especially Cynthia Perella and Marcia Clark, for being loving listeners and encouragers throughout the entire process. My siblings, Marilyn, Jim, and Billy, for prayers and loving encouragement. My daughters, Liz and Cate, whose love, prayers, notes, and moral support carried me forward.

My husband, Ambrose—my rock, my solid ground—for precise and practical help with editing, but more importantly for his abiding love, staunch support, and spiritual companionship on this journey.

And to the Lord, who inspired me with the idea for this project and graced me with the gifts to make it happen, I am humbly grateful.

Maureen Murray

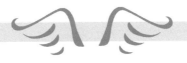

Introduction to Prayers

Although this volume contains specific prayers for each stage of the journey, you will find some degree of overlap, especially those prayers dealing with the emotional impact of breast cancer. I invite you to choose the prayers from any section that speak to your individual frame of mind and heart. The Table of Contents is structured with some degree of chronologic order, but many prayers, especially those in Part Five, actually apply to every section.

For prayers that required a gender reference, some are written as masculine and some as feminine, rather than using the more cumbersome he/she. You also may notice that each prayer contains references to thanksgiving for blessings already received. This is intentional and reflects my belief that gratitude—even in the face of great adversity—helps to foster a state of calmness and quiet perspective.

Part One:
A Journey You Did
Not Choose to Take

*"Fear not, for I am with you; do
not look anxiously about you, for I am
Your God."*

— Isaiah 41:10

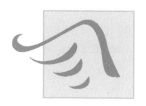

While Waiting for Pathology Results

Loving God, I reach out to You. The waiting is so difficult, and I am afraid. My emotions have shifted up and down, sideways, and inside out. My energy is scattered in a dozen directions, spiraling and speculating, twisting and turning. One minute I am overcome with anxiety, and the next minute I tell myself, and actually *believe*, that everything will be fine. I am so consumed with fatigue and worry that it is hard to concentrate on the routine tasks of the day.

Sometimes I forget for a few minutes that my cells are being examined at this very moment, and that the outcome could alter my life. Suddenly I remember, and uncertainty floods my mind with such fear that I feel cold all over. I remind myself that the situation is beyond my control, and the only thing to do now is to place myself in Your compassionate care.

The child in me wants to bargain with You and promise that I will make positive changes if I do not have cancer. I want to say, "Give me another chance to use my gifts and my time wisely, and I will not let You down." Then I realize that I do not need bad news or big scares to bring me closer to You. So as I wait for my results, help me to pause, be patient, and become more aware of Your presence.

At this very moment, I surrender my concerns—completely, utterly, totally—to Your loving protection. Sometimes it is hard for me to relinquish control, but that is what I wish to do. Please carry my fears for me so I can conserve my strength to cooperate with treatment, if it is required. Whatever the outcome, I know that You are my companion in every endeavor, challenge, or concern, and that You are with me now as I wait.

You may wish to turn to page 142 for the meditation "Place Your Cares on the Altar of God."

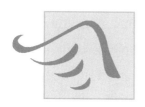

When the Diagnosis Is Breast Cancer

Lord, gather me to Yourself for consolation and strength. I have just heard news that frightens me to my core. When my doctor told me I have breast cancer, I felt like the diagnosis was being delivered to someone else. I asked questions and attempted to absorb the answers, but my mind could not grasp the information. I am stunned and numbed by the enormity of this single and unquestionable fact: I have breast cancer. My mind churns with more questions about treatments and prognosis, and I turn to You to guide my spirit through this storm.

You have been present with me when I heard other upsetting things—large or small—my entire life. You infused me with Your loving strength when I needed it most to deal with upsetting and even devastating news. Never have I spoken Your name that You did not rush to my aid and remain by my side. My gratitude for Your faithfulness and constancy is profound and heartfelt.

Hear my voice, loving Lord, as I call out again. Please walk with me again over rocky terrain, and extend Your arm to help me to keep my balance. Bless me with a heightened awareness of Your constant presence that calms my mind and spirit. Reassure me that we will face every moment of this challenge together, side by side, hand in hand.

You may wish to turn to page 146 for the meditation "Connecting With Your Angel."

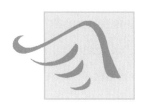

For Strength to See Beyond Fear

Blessed Source of Courage, fear consumes me at this moment, so with hope and trust in my heart, I turn to You for protection. My vision is clouded; I am having difficulty seeing past my anxiety. I know that my perspective has been affected by my illness, and now the future looks frightening and bleak. Instead of visualizing favorable outcomes, I see possibilities of more hurdles, treatments, and an uncertain prognosis. My stomach tightens, my shoulders tense, and my spirit sinks.

Lord, I have been afraid before, and when I talked to You, I felt serenity return to my soul. Your reply was swift and sure. Your constancy and acceptance have always restored my faith in the future.

Read the concern on my face and in my heart. In the comfort of Your love, I pour out the anxieties that stifle me and beg that my soul be restored to stillness. Strengthen me, Lord, to walk this challenging journey free of fear and dread. I ask that You gently release me from my concerns and bolster my spirit with peace. In Your everlasting goodness, renew my confidence to face any of life's setbacks with You at my side.

You may wish to turn to page 146 for the meditation "Connecting With Your Angel."

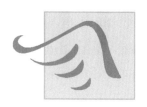

Before Telling Your Partner

Lord of Companionship, let me feel Your presence as I face the sensitive task of sharing my diagnosis with my partner. During our years together, we have witnessed and weathered many changes. I dread the prospect of inflicting anxiety and pain on the person with whom I share a relationship that encompasses our history and our hopes.

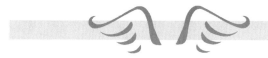

When Your Relationship Is Solid

_____ has enriched my life immeasurably. I am heartily thankful for the precious love that brings meaning and purpose to each day. Our enduring bond strengthens my resolve to face my fear with courage and look to a brighter future. Please grant me the wisdom to choose the right words to cushion this news with caring. Above all, bless me with the ability to express both my gratitude for our love and for my faith, that together with You and our doctors, we will triumph over this challenge.

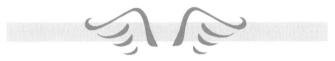

When Your Relationship Is Strained

_____'s presence in my life grew from expectations of joy but became difficult through the years. Give me the grace to withhold judgment and to remember the good that drew us together. Bless my partner with the generosity of spirit to rise above our differences and treat me with kindness during this time of stress and fear. Please grant me the wisdom to convey this news in a way that brings out the best in both my partner and myself.

You may wish to turn to page 153 for the meditation "Seeking Solid Ground."

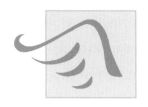

Before Telling Your Children

Heavenly Father, I dread telling my children that I have cancer, and I ask for Your loving guidance. I have rehearsed the words in my mind many times, but I still cannot find the right way to share this news. You have generously guided me to speak well-chosen words to my children on many occasions. Now I need Your compassionate help more than ever.

Young Children

Lord, you know that these precious and innocent children will believe anything I tell them about my health. Please give me the wisdom to share just enough so they will understand that I need time to rest. Help me to refrain from telling them too much. Guide me to answer their questions with truthfulness that is tempered with a loving awareness of their vulnerability. They are so young and they need protection from unnecessary fear. Help to provide me with insight and wisdom as I prepare for this sensitive task. Please help me to search for the best time and the right words to share this news with the cherished children You have entrusted to my care.

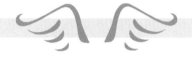

Older Children

Dear God, my heart aches at the prospect of telling my children I have cancer. I know their peace of mind will be terribly shaken. I am concerned that they will fear the worst because they have heard stories at school about other parents who had cancer. Help me to find the right moment in our busy lives, a little space when no one needs to write a paper or hurry to an activity. Inspire me with words that balance the reality of my situation with the sense of safety that my children still desperately need. Remind me that I do not have to hide all my anxiety, and let me show them that fear is natural and can be managed with optimism and faith. Grant me awareness that their fear may manifest itself as difficult behavior, and please give me the strength to be as patient and loving as I can.

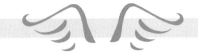

Adult Children

Lord, I know that my children will be saddened and scared by this news. They are adults with lives of their own, yet they are still my children no matter how old they are, and I know they will be fearful. Bless me with the gift of good judgment so that I may share with them my concerns without frightening them unnecessarily. If they have suggestions about my medical care, grant me the gift of an open mind to consider their input and a grateful heart that they care about me so deeply. My head says they have had experience with setbacks, but my heart knows that anything that threatens their mother will upset them. Inspire me with words that will inform, but not overwhelm, and let me deliver them with quiet reassurance.

You may wish to turn to page 150 for the meditation "Wrap Your Children in a Quilt of God's Love."

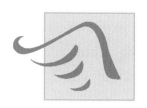

To Find the Right Surgeon

Eternal Healer, I am facing the challenging task of choosing a breast cancer surgeon, and there are so many factors to consider. I need someone with excellent skills who is focused and precise. I want a surgeon who is knowledgeable and open-minded about all the options and who will guide me without pressuring me. I am searching for someone who is willing to acknowledge my fear and treat me with dignity and respect.

In Your boundless generosity, You have led researchers to new treatments that prolong life and bring hope. You have inspired my trusted friends and family to search out recommendations for excellent surgeons. I am grateful to feel Your guiding hand on my shoulder as I take the next step.

I ask for Your loving guidance in this important decision. You are familiar with all my wants and needs. Please lead me to the surgeon who will recommend the procedure that is right for me. If my first appointment leaves me feeling unsettled and uncertain, grant me the courage to heed my inner voice and seek another opinion. Let me experience a trusting connection with my surgeon, and a spirit of mutual liking and respect so that I may cooperate fully with the procedure in mind, body, and spirit. Grant that You and my doctor and I become staunch allies on my healing journey.

You may wish to turn to page 169 for the meditation "Staying on Course."

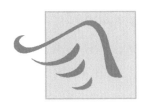

While in the Waiting Room

Lord of Serenity, the diagnosis of cancer makes waiting so much more difficult. Help me to remain calm and prayerful while I pass the time before seeing the physician to whom I have entrusted my care. Remain close to me as I sit on this chair, in this waiting room, at this moment. Remind me that this time of waiting is what I choose it to be: either a bother or an unexpected chance to think and pray for my loved ones and those who have been instrumental in my care. Give me the perspective to see that an opportunity for good may arrive disguised as an inconvenience. Bless me with patience as I sift through the maze of appointments and strive to fit them into the busyness of my daily life.

Thank you for the compassionate companionship and enduring support You have bestowed on me thus far in my journey. I lift up my grateful spirit to acknowledge the abundant grace I have received to help me face this challenge.

Please be a constant presence in the examining room as my doctor draws on Your healing gifts to diagnose and treat me. Guide him to bring forth his vast stores of hard-earned knowledge, and open his heart to my questions so that we may enter into a partnership of healing. Please tell him of my need to feel that he has adequate time to address my concerns without being rushed. If we are unable to create a positive relationship, please lead me to another physician with whom I can unite my healing energy and intent. Dear Lord, thank you for waiting with me. I breathe so much easier knowing that You are here.

You may wish to turn to page 142 for the meditation "Place Your Cares on the Altar of God."

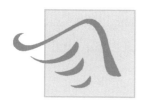

To Keep the Statistics in Perspective

Lord, You gave us the ability to quantify our world in order to understand it. We know how to plan and when to plant. We know how to predict weather and how to measure the food that sustains us. We can determine how much paint covers a wall, and we can calculate how to explore the reaches of the solar system. We can predict the probability that a cancer drug or treatment will be successful.

Sometimes the numbers sustain me, and sometimes they scare me. When I read projections about survival rates, they remind me that some women do not survive. When numbers are in my favor, I usually feel optimistic and confident. When the odds are not as favorable, I remind myself that numbers are only guidelines and not gospel truth.

But sometimes, in the quiet moments of the day or the stillness of night, the statistics seize a corner of my mind, and they nag like a persistent child who wants to be noticed. They create unwelcome mental chatter that distracts me from my work or sleep and causes me anxiety.

Loving God, remind me that statistics cannot measure the impact of faith or the healing power of prayer. I know that numbers cannot put a value on the will to survive and thrive. Plant firmly in my mind the absolute truth that You are the only one who knows the future, and if I spend my precious moments worrying about numbers, I am taking valuable time from my family, friends, and You. Enlighten me with perspective so that I may serve You with a calm sense of purpose and joy.

You may wish to turn to page 162 for the meditation "Seeing the Big Picture."

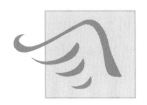

For the Wisdom to Make Correct Medical Choices

God of Knowledge and Insight, there are many decisions facing me as I begin the journey of breast cancer treatment. Many loving and kind people have shared recommendations and suggestions, and I am gathering and exploring options. There is so much to consider, I am struggling to keep from feeling overwhelmed with all the resources and information.

You have generously provided me with the ability to sift through alternatives and select a favorable plan of action. I have prayed for guidance about decisions, and Your response has been sure and steady, a flame illuminating the correct path. I am grateful for the times You have inspired me when I faced difficult choices. Please surround me with Your divine direction once again, and remain with me while I regain my footing.

Choosing the best physician and treatment requires so much more than facts; it calls for wisdom. I humbly ask You to inspire me to make the correct treatment decisions as I plan my care. Please bless me with a keen grasp of the details, and enable me to choose with certainty and confidence, not looking back to ruminate or second-guess. With You as my compass, I trust that my path will be clear because it is illuminated by Your love.

You may wish to turn to page 163 for the meditation "Open Your Heart to Wisdom."

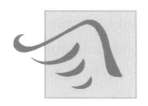

When You Are a Single Mother

Loving Father, I gaze deeply into the eyes of my precious children, and I want to weep. They need and love me so much that the prospect of anything happening to me floods my soul with sadness. Their lives would be split apart without me to provide words of reassurance, hugs of comfort and pride, practical help, and most of all, endless, unconditional love. I am the only parent they have from day to day, and I suffer with anxiety that my health could become worse.

You have parented me with constancy and unconditional love from the first day of my life. You gave me Your undivided attention every time I turned to You with challenges and concerns. When I asked for Your support, You responded with abundance and compassion. I am humbly grateful.

Now I entreat You as a parent to understand and soothe my fears about my children. Inspire me with the right words when I need to reassure them. Protect me from my concerns, and calm my troubled spirit so I may better focus on healing. Please create in me a sense of quiet purpose as I add a regimen of treatment to the many responsibilities and tasks of being a single mother. Restore me to wholeness of the body, mind, and spirit so that I may guide my children to become shining reflections of Your love. I surrender my cares and ask for Your loving comfort and reassurance.

You may wish to turn to page 150 for the meditation "Wrap Your Children in a Quilt of God's Love."

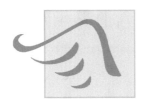

When You Are a Young Single Woman With Breast Cancer

Lord of Gentleness, I am heartsick. The news that I have breast cancer overwhelms me with shock and grief. I am so young to deal with this uncertainty and fear. My whole life is ahead of me, and I have such hopes and expectations for the future. What will happen to my plans for an exciting career and loving family of my own? I always assumed that I could make my dreams come true if I worked hard and lived a good life. I feel shattered into jagged pieces of sadness, anger, and fear, and I am struggling to put myself together again.

You have always been there for me when I called upon You. Even when I overload my schedule and do not give You much attention, You still respond to my pleas for help and surround me with Your loving presence. I am grateful for the rich blessings of Your protection and love. Please do not fail me now in this hour of desperate need.

I beg You to hear my prayer. Please ease my raging fear. Help me to regain a sense of calmness as I go forward to learn about what I must do to restore my health. Grant me the strength to endure the treatments with patience and hope and to cope with the emotional trauma of the diagnosis with courage and optimism. Reassure me that I will once again know peace of mind. When I falter, let me feel the reassuring touch of Your hand on mine and know beyond doubt that You have gathered me to Your heart.

You may wish to turn to page 142 for the meditation "Place Your Cares on the Altar of God."

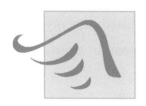

For Grandmothers With Breast Cancer

Heavenly Creator of Generations, I look at my beautiful grandchildren and I long to remain vital and healthy for them. The thought of being weakened by breast cancer and unable to enjoy the pleasures of being a grandmother saddens my heart. I would not want them to be sad or scared at seeing their grandma being sick. Even though I strive to remain optimistic, sometimes a lurking fear creeps into my mind, quietly puts down roots, and remains an unwelcome guest.

My delight in my grandchildren makes my heart sing out with joy. They bring sunshine and freshness and magic into my life, and I love them so much. I am grateful for the privilege of knowing and loving my children's children.

Please shine Your healing light upon me and restore my strength and enthusiasm. Let me lavish my love on my grandchildren and savor the joy of the present moment, unfettered by fears about the future. Allow me to serve as an example for them, courageously facing medical treatments with a spirit of hope and renewal. Grant that the abundance my grandchildren bring to my life will grow even greater in the shining light of Your love.

You may wish to turn to page 149 for the meditation "Seeking Peace of Mind and Heart."

Part Two: Gathering Your Strength for Traveling Through Uncertain Times

"Be strong and courageous; do not be terrified; do not be discouraged, for the Hand of God will be with you wherever you go."

— Joshua 1:9

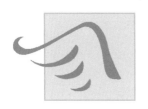

For Your Surgeon

God of all Protection, lovingly guide the skillful hands of my surgeon as she performs this procedure so vital to my healing. Provide her with the gifts of concentration and meticulous precision to remove any growth that is harmful to my health and well-being. Focus her mind on the satisfaction in her work and on the positive intent that my body will respond and recover quickly from this surgery. Fill her heart with gratitude for the healing gifts you have so generously bestowed and which she has worked so hard to develop.

Thank you for guiding me to connect with this surgeon in whom I have placed my complete trust. I am grateful that we have agreed on the best plan for my recovery from the medical challenge that lies before me.

Magnificent Healer, please guide my surgeon in the operating room. Let her instill in the entire surgical team a spirit of collaboration and genuine caring for me as they minister to my needs. Surround her with the grace of knowing that she honors You in a profound way by being the best surgeon and person she can be.

You may wish to turn to page 167 for the meditation "Surround Caregivers With Grace."

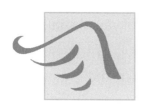

For Concerns About Anesthesia

Eternal God of Consciousness, the prospect of anesthesia frightens me. Hearing my diagnosis of breast cancer and accepting that I need surgery greatly challenged my spirit and serenity. With Your compassionate help, I am becoming calm and confident about the outcome. But anesthesia scares me at a level that defies logic. The thought of being unconscious, powerless, and vulnerable fills me with anxiety.

Every night, You protect me as I drift into sleep, oblivious to the world's cares and my own worries. Each morning, I awaken and gradually return to being alert and aware. I am grateful for the natural ebb and flow of my day's activity and rest. Let me think of anesthesia as a sleeping and waking to restore health, a grace-filled and blessed forgetting.

Let Your light shine on my anesthesiologist for the duration of my surgery. Keep her mind free of all distractions as she monitors my condition with vigilance and care. Allow my body to tolerate the anesthesia easily, and awaken me to gratitude that all has gone well. I know that You will be standing next to me in the recovery room, and this gives me courage and strength to surrender my fear.

You may wish to turn to page 149 for the meditation "Seeking Peace of Mind and Heart."

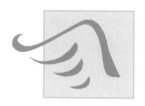

The Night Before Surgery

Lord of Courage, the time is close, and my mind is consumed with anxiety about my surgery tomorrow. I want it to be over, but I do not want to go through it. My faith in my surgeon eases some of my fears, but I worry about anesthesia, lymph nodes, pathology, and prognosis. I dread a restless night and that waking sensation of something being wrong.

I know that with Your soothing encouragement, I have faced fear before. When I was afraid, You showed me how to go deep inside and tap into strength that was steady and strong. With the assurance of Your constant presence, I knew I could face anything. Thank you deeply and humbly for always being there for me.

Bless me with a brave heart and optimistic outlook as I prepare for tomorrow. Let me visualize the entire operating room illuminated with the unwavering light of Your love. Bless me with some measure of restful sleep tonight so that I am strong in body and spirit for the surgery. Please stand watch over me tonight and allow me to experience Your loving protection as my first waking thought. Good night, Lord. Your closeness gives me courage and peace.

You may wish to turn to page 147 for the meditation "Cloak Yourself With Courage."

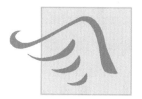

Before Leaving for the Hospital for Surgery

Most Compassionate Lord, the unknown looms large in front of me as I head to the hospital for my surgery. The knots in my stomach have tied themselves with the intensity of a dedicated scout. Although my head tells me that everything will go well, my cold hands reflect the anxiety that lies deep within my heart. I know I am not reacting in a normal way to things my loved ones are saying to me. It feels like I have grown a protective shell to shield my spirit until the worst is over.

I could not do this without you, Lord. I know You are here, and I feel Your love and kindness. I am deeply reassured that I will never be alone. Thank you for removing my sense of isolation and reassuring me that You and I will go through the hospital doors together.

Please bless me with both calmness and courage as I collect myself before the surgery.

Shelter me under the protective arm of Your wondrous love, and allow me to breathe deeply and freely with renewed confidence in the outcome of my surgery. I bow to You and place myself in Your tender care at this moment and for all the days of my life. We are leaving now, Lord. Take my hand. Your presence makes me strong for the journey.

You may wish to turn to page 147 for the meditation "Cloak Yourself With Courage."

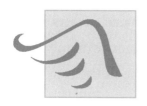

In the Surgical Holding Area

Lord, I feel so vulnerable. I am lying here in a hospital gown with an IV in my arm and everyone else is standing, fully clothed, going about their business. I know they are trying to be kind to me (and if they are not, grant me the perspective not to take it personally), but I am still struggling to reduce my fear and increase my faith that all will go well. Lessen my emotional resistance to this procedure and allow me to surrender my safety to You and the medical caregivers You have provided for me.

You already have blessed me with the benevolence of Your faithful and everlasting love as I walked through the steps leading up to this moment. You have surrounded me with the fortress of Your guidance and protection, and for this I am grateful.

In a few minutes, I will be totally in the care of others. Let them be free of distraction so they can use their skills to care for me with clear minds and loving hearts. I know You will be in the operating room with me during the entire procedure, so please let a feeling of complete trust wash over me now as I wait to be called. Thank you, dear Lord, for understanding my fears and reassuring me of your Faithful Presence. You are in charge now. Hear my heartfelt plea for Your protection, and open my spirit to the pathway of Your peace.

You may wish to turn to page 158 for the meditation "Activate Your Healing Energy."

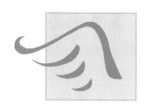

To Be Said With Your Surgeon

This prayer is shorter than the others because busy operating room schedules sometimes require that your pre-op meeting with your surgeon is brief. Also, ask your surgeon ahead of time if she will say a short prayer with you before you are taken to surgery. This could prevent you from being disappointed or upset if you surprise her with this request and the answer is no. If your surgeon prefers not to participate in prayer with you, try not to feel discouraged or take it personally. Simply substitute "I" for "we" and "me/my" for "our/us" and offer this additional prayer for yourself. The Lord perfectly understands your intent.

Divine Lord, we humbly ask Your blessing as we prepare to enter the operating room. Fill our hearts with positive thoughts about the process and outcome of the surgery. Remind us that You are the source of all healing, and hold us close to You now and throughout the procedure. Bless the entire surgical team as we work together to restore health and wholeness. Together we offer our gratitude and praise for Your faithful presence now and forever.

You may wish to turn to page 158 for the meditation "Activate Your Healing Energy."

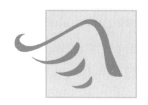

To Be Said for You While You Are in Surgery

Divine Physician, please bless _____ _____ (your name) while she is undergoing surgery. Instill in her surgical team a sense of loving kindness and sacred duty to perform at their highest levels of sharply focused skill. Free their minds of all thoughts except those that further the progress of the surgery and generate healing energy. Inspire her team to only make comments that are positive, uplifting, and nurturing.

Guide _____ as she is under anesthesia to connect with the powerful, internal healing forces that You have lovingly created to restore health. You have blessed us with Your everlasting presence, so let her deeply feel the comfort of Your closeness and know that she is cherished and protected during her surgery.

Lord, please let her feel the restorative power of the tender prayers I offer for her at this moment. I know that prayer transcends time and space, and in Your infinite wisdom, You have granted us this gift for joining ourselves to You and to each other. Let her feel the depth of my care as I offer these prayers for the success of her surgery. Please accept my humble gratitude that You have heard this heartfelt petition.

You may wish to turn to page 167 for the meditation "Surround Caregivers With Grace."

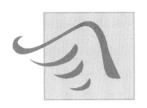

For Your Nurses

Compassionate God, I know that many nurses labor long hours and shoulder enormous responsibilities. So first, I offer this prayer that they will be given some respite from the ongoing challenges that deplete their energy. Shower them with plentiful blessings to restore and rejuvenate their spirits, because they are indeed the heart of every hospital, the gentle guardians of the healing process.

I am deeply grateful for their dedication to healing and appreciate the many kindnesses they have shown me already. Please grant them an extra minute to hold my hand, pat my arm and reassure me that everything will be fine, or help me accept news that is difficult to hear. Let them respond with empathy to my anxiety about these unfamiliar procedures. Direct them to look at me with eyes that connect to the concerns deep within my soul.

Lord, please provide them the rest they need after a long day of caring for others, as well as me. Create in their lives some time and space so they can fill up the well that caregivers draw from each day. Protect them from "running on empty" by helping them to juggle the many tasks in their lives so they may continue to minister with tenderness and loving care. Surround them with Your mercy and goodness as they enter the hospital each day to serve You and the patients in their care.

You may wish to turn to page 167 for the meditation "Surround Caregivers With Grace."

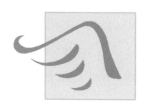

Thanksgiving After Surgery

(To be said by you when you are able and for you by a loved one when you are in the recovery room.)

Lord of Protection, the surgery is finished, and my relief is great. I feel like I can finally exhale the breath I have been holding since this process began and focus on the next step on the journey to health.

I know that Your healing presence in the operating room served as a guiding beacon for my surgeon and the entire team. You, who steady the hand of all who perform surgery, stood a faithful watch to ensure that all would be well. My thankfulness fills and overflows my spirit, and I joyfully praise Your Holy Name.

As this healing journey continues, please remain close so that we may draw each breath together, joined by the bond of Your compassion and love. Bless the surgical team with quiet concentration as they complete the day's work and with restful sleep as they prepare for tomorrow. I am awed by Your never-ending concern for my loved ones and me. I offer humble thanks for Your loving protection and presence.

You may wish to turn to page 167 for the meditation "Surround Caregivers With Grace."

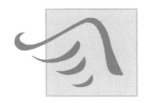

If You Learn That You Need Chemotherapy

Precious Lord, I feel so deflated to learn that I need chemotherapy. When I heard the news, I felt my energy sink and my anxiety rise. I had been hoping that my lymph nodes would be negative and the tumor small enough that chemo would not be required. Now, I am facing months of anxiety, fatigue, and uncertainty about what to do and how to plan my daily life.

In my head, I am relieved and grateful that my surgery is successfully completed and I am recovering well. In my heart, I am disappointed, sad, and scared. I desperately wanted the whole process to be much simpler.

Please grant me the courage to endure whatever treatments will make me whole and strong again. Gently remind me that side effects are short-lived and bearable. Reassure me that You have given me the strength for this next step, and that I need only to go deep in my soul and find what is already there. I know that I can endure inconvenience and discomfort as long as I am not alone. I take great comfort in Your loving presence.

You may wish to turn to page 143 for the meditation "Direct Treatments to Their Target."

Part Three: Continuing Your Pilgrimage Toward Wholeness and Healing

"Let us run with endurance the race that is set before us."

—Hebrews 12:1

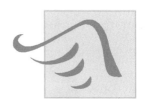

To Accept the Changes in Your Body

Divine Sculptor, sometimes the changes in my body sadden and upset me. The prospect of living with constant reminders of breast cancer discourages me and saps my energy. In the worst moments, I see my body as compromised and damaged. In better moments, I simply see scars that have healed well and are a testimony to a skilled surgeon and the advances of medicine. During these times, I am thankful that my condition was diagnosed and that I have moved forward.

In Your master blueprint for all of creation, You lovingly formed the human body. I am awed by the complex array of systems working in harmony. My gratitude is deep for the years of vitality and health You lovingly bestowed on me.

Please help me come to terms with change and accept that my body is different now. Remind me that in the limits of the body, I may discover wholeness of spirit. Paint the broad picture for me with the loving brushstrokes of Your perspective. My lack of acceptance consumes energy that is better used for more productive thoughts. I know that the human condition is imperfect in both body and behavior, and everything about us is precious to You. Dearest Lord, help me to translate this awareness from the words in my head to the language of my heart.

You may wish to turn to page 145 for the meditation "Create a Veil of Love for Your Head."

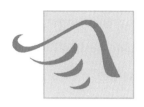

Before Seeing Your Oncologist

Heavenly Father, the word *oncologist* spreads through the corners of my mind, and I feel stunned. How is it that an appointment with an oncologist stares back from my calendar? Those dates should be written on somebody else's life planner, not mine. So often we assume that an accident or a disease will happen to the next person, so when it appears unbidden in our own lives, we are shocked. I am still feeling that jolt of harsh reality as I prepare for this visit.

You were there with me during the news of the diagnosis and the trauma of the surgery. I relied on Your support and reassurance, and You never left me for an instant. My gratitude for Your enduring support speaks from deep within my soul.

I am standing ready to put my foot on the next step. My concerns about the treatments flood me with new apprehension, and I humbly beg You to slow the beating of my anxious heart. Help me to lean forward into this new phase with total trust in its success. Grant that I will have minimal side effects. Bless my oncologist with abundant wisdom and expertise to choose the most effective regimen to restore my vitality and health.

You may wish to turn to page 145 for the meditation "Create a Veil of Love for Your Head."

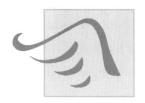

Before Radiation Treatment

Lord of Light, as I prepare for radiation, bless me with an appreciation for the wonders of Your creation. Reduce my fear about the treatment by reminding me that radiation already occurs throughout Your bountiful universe in rock formations and even in sunshine. When I know this healing tool occurs naturally, I can appreciate it more and manage my concerns better.

Bless me with a calm resolve and an optimistic spirit as I enter this stage of my care. Activate the deep wisdom of my body so that the radiation reaches its destination swiftly and surely. Fill my surrounding cells with vitality and energy so they may stay strong, and form a shield between the margins of cancer and my healthy tissue.

Help me to visualize radiation as a healing light that You have endowed with special powers to restore. Grant me the wisdom to view my body's need for additional rest as a marker along my personal road to recovery. Please provide me with the vision to view these days of radiation with gratitude for the wonders of technology. I praise You for directing the minds of medical researchers to harness such a potent force. I submit myself to Your loving care as I choose to undergo this positive and healing treatment.

You may wish to turn to page 143 for the meditation "Direct Treatments to Their Target."

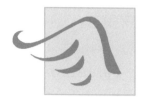

Before a Chemotherapy Session

Sublime Healer, You know I have great anxiety about chemotherapy. I dread any treatment that puts toxic chemicals into my body in order to cure me. I know that many women have remissions after their treatments, but I also have heard about the many side effects of chemo, and I am worried.

You have created the universe and all the elements needed to formulate these potent medicines. You have blessed scientists with the knowledge and skill to create treatments that prolong lives and alleviate suffering. With loving benevolence, You have provided the raw materials that my caregivers use to help restore my good health. Please place Your loving hands on theirs as they prepare and administer the chemotherapy that I have chosen to undergo.

As You guide my medical team in the management of my care, please direct each of my cells to respond to this treatment in the best way possible. Let my body use its innate wisdom to gain maximum benefit with minimum side effects. If I experience hair loss, help me to put it in the larger context of my healing and to keep in mind that it is temporary and shall pass. If side effects occur, guide me to discuss them with my doctor, for perhaps they are signs that the medications are working. Remind me that rest will help to restore my health.

Gracious God, let these carefully chosen drugs do their work in an accurate and efficient way so that I may use my renewed energy and strength to glorify Your holy name.

You may wish to turn to pages 143 and 145 for the meditations "Direct Treatments to Their Target" and "Create a Veil of Love for Your Head."

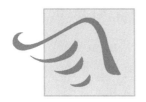

For the Strength to Get Through the Day

Lord of Infinite Energy, I am weary. Anxiety, appointments, and treatments are sapping my strength. I am so far behind that I stopped keeping track. It is an enormous struggle to put one foot in front of the other as I go about my daily routines. I feel like I am dragging myself through the day with the major goal of going back to sleep. Morning comes before I am rested, then it starts all over again.

Please bless me with little bursts of energy so I can accomplish a few small things, then direct me to rest and restore my body and spirit. Guide me to release my concerns about being useful and productive and to direct my energy toward wholeness and healing. Instill in me a greater acceptance of my needs and limitations. Send into my life generous and compassionate people to help with practical concerns until I emerge from this period of fatigue. A ride to an appointment, a dinner dropped off at my home, a carpool for my children, _____ (mention your own needs) would be deeply appreciated right now. Thank you for hearing my requests with such care and compassion.

Lord, do not let me be proud. If I do not receive offers of help, then grant me the humility to ask. You and I both know there are many loving people out there who would not consider my simple requests an imposition. Remind me that by offering them the chance to help me in my time of need I am, in fact, giving them two important gifts: the opportunity to praise and glorify You through service and the satisfied heart that follows acts of kindness.

I pray that this time of fatigue will pass easily. In the meantime, I ask You to provide me with energy for what is really important and the wisdom to let go of the rest.

You may wish to turn to page 165 for the meditation "Search for Sun in Gray Skies."

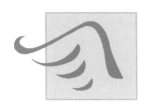

When It Is Difficult to Eat

Heavenly Provider, it is such a challenge to eat; yet I know I need nourishment to heal. The sights and smells of delicious meals I used to enjoy make me feel queasy and sick. I am aware that I must eat, and when nothing appeals to me, I feel anxious and even guilty that I am not doing all I can to support my healing. Loving family and friends encourage me and prepare special menus to tempt my appetite, but I have little interest in food.

In the best of times, I have asked Your divine blessing on abundant meals I shared with loving family and friends. You provided me with a rich array of foods and a healthy appetite to savor them. Your endless generosity fills me with gratitude for all that I have received. I am especially thankful right now for the dinners that others so generously provide for my family.

Please grant me the perspective to endure this time with perseverance and grace. When I am inclined to complain, remind me that there have been many happier and enjoyable times at my table in the past, and they await me in the future. Bless me with the fortitude and patience to keep trying different foods and to find some that work for the time being. Above all, let Your eternal presence and love continue to nourish my body, mind, and spirit. Your divine sustenance feeds me and gives me renewed hope.

You may wish to turn to page 165 for the meditation "Search for Sun in Gray Skies."

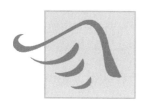

When You Must Take Ongoing Medication

Steadfast and Enduring Lord, with Your help, the surgery and treatments are behind me. As I begin this next step of daily medication, I have concerns about the safety and long-term effects. I wonder if the medication will agree with me, and if it will be effective in doing its job of preventing a recurrence. I have read and heard information that troubles me and have weighed the consequences and made the decision to go forward. Sometimes disturbing second thoughts creep into my mind.

I have placed my complete trust in You on every step of this disquieting medical journey that thrust itself into my life. You were staunch, compassionate, and loving at each milestone, from diagnosis to follow-up care. When I was too weary to walk, You carried me. When I was uncertain, You were my strength. How blessed I felt to know that Your loving arms enfolded and protected me always.

Please ease my concerns about the daily medication. Direct it to perform its job precisely and well. Let me focus on its healing effects and not on its risks. Reassure me that this final stage of my healing improves my chances for vitality and good health, and encourage me to stay on track. By Your divine direction, please allow me to tolerate the medication, and minimize any side effects so that I have renewed energy to love and serve You.

You may wish to turn to page 169 for the meditation "Staying on Course."

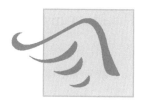

When Your Children Are Sad and Concerned About You

Compassionate Father, my heart aches with sadness when I calculate the toll my cancer takes on my children. They look at me with knowing eyes: the older ones aware that I struggle with my own fears and fatigue; the younger ones simply needing reassurance that Mom is okay. I long to tell them with certainty that all will be well, and things will be back to normal before they know it. They keep tabs on me with questions about how I feel, what the doctor said, and what is next in the process. I realize they yearn to regain some control in their lives, and I desperately wish I could provide it for them.

I know that hidden underneath this challenge is the opportunity for my children to become more resilient and compassionate. I know, too, that You already have been the sacred rock they stood on when they faced other setbacks in their lives. I am grateful for these blessings.

With every breath and every beat of my heart, I ask that You comfort and support my children. Their concern for me depletes their energy and joy; it leads them down the blind path of fear. Open their hearts to happiness again, and let them laugh with the same abandon as before. Envelop them in the cloak of Your loving protection, and assure them that this darkness will soon be followed by glorious dawn.

You may wish to turn to page 150 for the meditation "Wrap Your Children in a Quilt of God's Love."

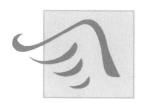

When You Are in Pain

Lord, I turn to You in my pain and beg Your comfort and release. Cancer is taking a heavy toll on my body and spirit, and I am struggling to be strong. My body aches, and my soul is filled with sadness and fear. I am grappling with the realization that my peace of mind may never completely mend. I yearn for my former pain-free life of vitality and good health.

You have encouraged us to turn to You when we suffer from discouragement and pain. I beseech You to bear witness to my pain. Grant me the courage to endure it well and the wisdom to accept medication from my caregivers so that I do not cause unnecessary suffering for them or me. I know that You are with me even now as I stand before You, and I am grateful for Your faithful companionship. It gives me hope and connects me to my inner strength.

Please rest a while with me now and soothe the hurts of my body and spirit. Whisper words that inspire me to direct my thoughts to Your loving presence. Grant me Your compassion as a soothing balm for the wounds I now endure. Let my suffering teach me greater sympathy for all who suffer, and remind me that it is only human to sometimes feel overwhelmed. Gather me close to You so I may rise above the pain to glorify Your name.

You may wish to turn to page 159 for the meditation "Feel the Hand of God Upon Your Face."

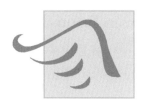

When Treatment Seems Never Ending

God of Everlasting Patience, this whole process seems like it is dragging on forever: the doctor visits, diagnostic procedures, waiting for results, surgery, follow-up treatments, medications, the changes I needed to make in my daily life and schedule. When will my life be my own again? The months of treatment are shifting my image of myself from healthy and vital to "cancer patient," words I still cannot believe apply to me.

Shower me with the blessing of endurance. Fill me with fortitude. Satisfy my longing for "normal" with a quiet persistence that helps me to look forward with vision and clarity. Remind me that there is an internal time schedule for the body's healing process, and my annoyance with its duration simply undermines the calm I wish to achieve. Tell me again to focus on my gratitude for how far I have come and for the outpouring of love from family and friends.

And, Dear Lord, here is my biggest request: Help me to reconsider my concept of time. Teach me to redefine it in terms of priority rather than productivity. Hush the chatter in my mind that continually pushes me to undertake another task. Speak gently into my ears of the need to cooperate fully with my treatment by remaining relaxed and unruffled. Remind me that nothing else—other than faithfulness to You—is more important than restoring my health. Let me use my energy to quiet my impatient spirit and cultivate a serene and grateful heart.

You may wish to turn to page 169 for the meditation "Staying on Course."

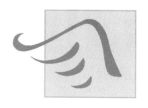

For Strength for Loved Ones

Caring Lord, I know my illness has a great impact on those I love. They share my anxiety about my progress and my prognosis. They worry about my treatments, my fatigue, my lack of appetite, and, most of all, my discouragement. They even try to make me laugh. They attempt to be cheerful around me, but sometimes I see the sadness and concern in their eyes, and my heart grows heavy.

How could I ever express my gratitude for the constancy of their love and support? How can I thank You enough for sending them to expand and enrich my life? I am indeed wealthy beyond measure with the kindness and care I receive from them and You.

Strengthen them, Lord. Give them respite from the emotional challenge of caring for me. Reassure them that they are doing the very best they can, and they can rely on You as a partner in healing. Grant them release from the fears that sap their spirits, and hope in the promise of brighter tomorrows. Please bless them with renewed energy, the relief of laughter, and the gift of restful sleep. Watch over them as gently and tenderly as they watch over me, and awaken them to the blessing of a lighter heart.

You may wish to turn to page 142 for the meditation "Place Your Cares on the Altar of God."

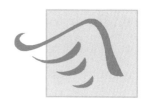

For Your Support Group

Blessed Encourager, the women in my support group are in very different places on their journey to healing. Some are anxious and fearful, others hopeful and confident. Some are outspoken and definite, others tentative and quiet. Yet every one of them has a sensitive and tender place in her spirit that was imprinted by cancer. Each woman shows her personal way of coping with a condition that fractured her life and challenged her to put it back together.

I thank You for connecting me to all of them. I know that I can learn from some and serve as a humble teacher to others. I am grateful for inspiration from those whose courage clearly shows. Let me respond with renewed compassion to those who dwell in fear.

Please infuse our support group with a spirit of sharing and caring so we may each contribute according to our gifts and needs. Allow us to find some blessed laughter in the midst of our anxiety. Like the miracle of sunshine and shadow, let us give and receive as we may, illuminating and absorbing radiance in return. Bless our leader as she manifests her gifts of listening and speaking with a gentle spirit. Grant each of us a deep and ongoing trust in Your everlasting presence as a member of our group.

You may wish to turn to page 167 for the meditation "Surround Caregivers With Grace."

Part Four: The Road Ahead

"Weave in faith and God will find the thread."

—Proverb

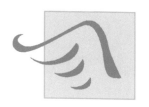

To Accept That Things Are Different

Precious and Perceptive God, You already know that deep within me, I am having trouble admitting a basic truth: Life is different now. My diagnosis of breast cancer marked a loss of innocence, an about-face in an image of myself as vital and healthy. The shock waves vibrate deep in my heart, casting about for a foothold while I swing back and forth between ignoring them and latching onto them. The news of cancer shattered my faith that my body could defend itself from invaders. It slammed into my peace of mind with a thud. The sense that life will never be the same wounds my spirit.

You already have been generous beyond measure in providing me with peace of mind about my health. When I took it for granted, I did not intend to be ungrateful but simply became immersed in the tasks of daily living. You gave me the ability to weather life's past changes and learn that with You by my side, I can handle anything. I am deeply grateful.

This is my heartfelt petition: please bless me with the inner strength to accept that although life is different, and certainly less secure, it does not need to be filled with anxiety. Ease my resistance to accepting the changes that cancer brings. Remind me that trying to cling to the past depletes my energy and diverts my attention from the process of healing. Help me to see with "new eyes" that the loss of security about the future can transform my appreciation of the present and its priceless gifts.

You may wish to turn to page 153 for the meditation "Seeking Solid Ground."

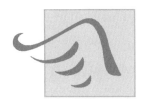

Survivor's Prayer of Thanksgiving

Gracious Giver of all Gifts, You have blessed me with magnificent abundance. In the majesty of Your eternal love, You have brought me through my fear and uncertainty to a place of deeper faith. When fatigue weighed me down, You restored me with renewed energy or carried me in Your arms. When my tasks overwhelmed me, You provided compassionate friends to help and inspired me to prioritize the urgent and to let go of the rest. When I was too frightened to feel anything, You loaned me Your heart.

Your unsurpassed bounty humbles me as never before. I stand before You, my heart filled with thanksgiving. My mind overflows with utter joy at being healthy again. I search for ways to express my gratitude that You have reawakened my vitality and joy.

Sustain in me the blessed relief and sweet happiness I feel at this moment. Remind me to share my blessings generously with other women by being a deep and compassionate friend and a source of information and comfort. Never let me forget that it is through Your shining grace that I endured and now flourish. Guide my steps as I search for opportunities to serve, share, listen, and learn. Above all, let me be ceaseless in my thanks and praise.

You may wish to turn to page 155 for the meditation "Sing a Song of Thanksgiving."

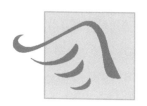

For the Courage to Change Your Life

Heavenly Source of Time, my experience with cancer has given me many hours to think. Sometimes I sit in waiting rooms or lie sleepless in bed and wonder what meaning I will take from this life-changing experience.

You have taught me that cancer is the fastest way to slow down—something I always expected to do when I grew older. I envisioned traveling to destinations that soothe my soul and taking in the sound of the surf or watching the sun's rays cast a glorious palette on the water. How clearly I pictured myself savoring a cup of steaming coffee while I organized the family photos I had stuffed into shoeboxes for years. I had a clear image of spending more time with family and friends, near and far, sharing old memories and creating new ones.

Thank you for teaching me that the future exists nowhere but in this moment. You have wiped away the clouds of self-deception from my eyes and revealed with stunning clarity the precious value of living in the present. You have given me the rare gift of perspective, the foundation upon which we build lives of satisfaction and purpose. I beg You for the strength to guard these lessons well, to make them a part of my being, and to set new priorities that nourish the treasures in my life.

Fill me with clarity that I may see the life you have in mind for me. Grant me the courage to claim the joy You have lovingly placed in my path and the wisdom to choose lasting change.

You may wish to turn to page 163 for the meditation "Open Your Heart to Wisdom."

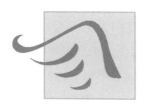

Prayer Before a Mammogram

Lord, deep inside I am worried about this mammogram. It brings back fearful memories of the procedure that uncovered the cancer in my breast. With my stomach in knots, I shiver with cold and fear while I wait to talk to the radiologist.

In the days and hours leading up to this checkup, please provide me with courage and draw me close to You. Hold my hand as a loving parent grasps the hand of a precious and frightened child, for I know that even in my vulnerability, I am a treasure in Your eyes. Soothe me with a soft voice that whispers, "It's all right. I am here." I am filled with gratitude for Your constant support since the day of my diagnosis and ask that You stand very close to me today.

I know that the outcome of this checkup will probably be fine. Surround me with hope and optimism for a future where I will praise Your name and appreciate the beauty of Your world. If I must face more medical challenges, I ask for the strength to be calm and clear-headed, trusting that You will remain close to me. Fill my lungs with Your very breath so that I may feel Your reassuring presence.

You may wish to turn to page 147 for the meditation "Cloak Yourself With Courage."

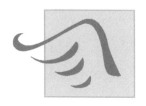

When You Have a Recurrence

Compassionate Lord, my cup of sadness overflows. My dreams of a cancer-free life have been shattered with the news of a recurrence. I am desperately struggling to deal with this news, but I am devastated. I keep thinking "Why me?" even though I know that same question also applies to all of the good things in my life. The prospect of more surgery and treatment overwhelms me with feelings of dread. I feel like my body ignored my efforts to lead a healthy life and, in a way, betrayed me. I feel vulnerable, dejected, angry, and afraid.

You sustained me through the first episode of breast cancer with Your constant presence. You provided me with the ultimate comfort of knowing that You understood, accepted, and loved me for my displays of both courage and fear. You surrounded me with generous and caring family and friends to sit with me, help me, and pray for me. I offer my deep gratitude for all You have done.

I turn to You again in this time that truly challenges my soul. Let my anxiety be replaced with Your comfort. Reach toward me, gently remove my burden, and place it on Your heavenly altar. Guard it for me until I feel stronger and more able to shoulder it. I beg You to be fearless for me when I am fearful and steady for me when I sway. Wrap Your loving arms around me, protect me from my fear, and assure me that I am always safe in Your presence.

You may wish to turn to page 142 for the meditation "Place Your Cares on the Altar of God."

Part Five:
For Any Time
You Need
Encouragement

"Be joyful in hope, patient in affliction, faithful in prayer."
—Romans 12:12

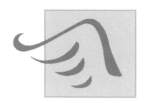

For Long, Dark Evenings

Lord, the growing darkness outside deepens the shadows in my heart. My worries grow larger as daylight fades and dusk turns into night. I cope with my fears better and feel stronger when I can see the sun. Please keep reminding me that You, the Source of all Light, are with me at every moment to ease my load and illuminate my path as I go forward on my healing journey.

I offer humble and heartfelt thanks for Your gift of brilliant light. Let the knowledge that it will faithfully return tomorrow sustain me through the evening, and bolster my spirits with trust.

Let me fill these long evening hours with positive thoughts and pleasant activities that distract me from my anxiety. Keep me company, and kindle in me the flame of Your love. When I lie down to restore my body and spirit for the challenges and tasks of tomorrow, grant me the comfort of knowing that the eyes of my soul can see Your blessed sunshine even in total darkness. May the light of Your love serve as my guiding beacon.

You may wish to turn to page 161 for the meditation "Call Forth Light in the Midst of Darkness."

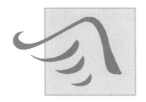

In the Middle of the Night (or When You Cannot Sleep)

Lord, these are the hardest hours to get through. When I awaken in the middle of the night, sometimes I am overcome with a fear that shakes my spirit and fills me with dread. I start to imagine the worst outcomes and create in my mind a future that is frightening and bleak. I know that in Your infinite wisdom and love, You created time for renewal, yet rest escapes me now, and the hours until daybreak seem long and lonely. Please help me to get through this night by focusing on the darkness as a time when I am free to be still in body and spirit.

Thank you for this time of respite from demands, responsibilities, and tasks. I am grateful for freedom from ringing phones, multiple messages, and countless requests. When I am not burdened with worry, I appreciate even more the soft stillness and quiet hush of night's shelter.

Now, as I try to quiet the beating of my restless heart, let me feel Your loving Presence so I know I am not alone. Let me hear Your voice in the deep silence of the night. Loving God, please wrap Your arms around me and let me rest my head on Your shoulder. Fill my spirit with the calmness that only You possess. Bear with me, and whisper to me again that You will always be with me. Precious Lord, stay with me through this night and, together, let us greet the dawn.

You may wish to turn to page 161 for the meditation "Call Forth Light in the Midst of Darkness."

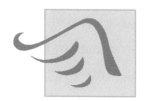

For the Strength to Put It Out of Your Mind for a While

It is always there, Lord. If it is not in the front of my mind, it is in the back. Whether I am going to work, running errands, or doing things around the house, something always reminds me of breast cancer. Sometimes it is an item in the newspaper, or I learn about someone else being newly diagnosed. Most upsetting is when I am at a party or in a restaurant, relaxed and enjoying myself, and an acquaintance approaches me with a well-meaning "How ARE you?" I force myself to respond pleasantly, while inside I wonder why they do not realize that I need to forget sometimes.

Thank you for the countless people who genuinely care about me. Let me remember that they ask out of concern, and remind me to keep in mind their good intentions. Help me to overlook those who ask out of curiosity. Give me the grace to answer them with the same kindness I would want to receive myself. Rather than considering their questions intrusive, remind me to let it go and remember the good times and the golden moments I have enjoyed.

Grant me a touch of forgetfulness. Sweep my mind clean of the word *cancer* with the broom of Your compassion. Grant me a brief reprieve—a mini-vacation from the awareness of cancer. After a break, I will return willingly to the reality of my life and concentrate on the steps I will take to become and remain well.

Lord, hopefully, in time, I will handle the reminders with greater ease, mentally acknowledging that I had cancer, then moving on. With Your grace, I pray that someday I will look back and say, "Yes, cancer changed my life, and some of the changes were positive."

You may wish to turn to page 149 for the meditation "Seeking Peace of Mind and Heart."

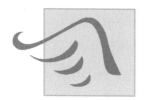

To Get Through the Holidays (and Other Special Occasions)

Lord of Celebration and Joy, my heart is not into holiday preparations this year. Either I am preoccupied with my medical treatment, or I simply do not have the mental or physical energy to focus on the festivities. I feel overwhelmed at the thought of shopping, wrapping, cleaning, cooking, and sending cards. For years, I have said that I wanted to simplify the holidays, and now that I have good reason to do that, I find myself wavering.

I ask You for strength. Bless me with the willpower to say a gracious "no" to the countless invitations, requests, and demands on my time. Remind me that by trying to please everyone, I ultimately will please no one, especially myself. Give me the resolve to hold firm to my decision to have simple holidays that revolve around family and friends, not glitter and gifts.

Let this be the year that I set the tone for the holidays to come. Thank you for the vivid mental pictures of gift exchanges that are heartfelt and not hectic and of relaxed family dinners with pleasant conversation. I visualize favorite traditional foods but not so many that the preparations become burdensome. I am especially grateful for my unwavering decision to accept more help this year.

Precious Lord, with Your help, I can create a simple celebration. Remind me that using my energy to prepare an extra dish or search for the perfect gift undermines my resolution to enjoy what matters most. Let Your light be a beacon to draw me to the true spirit of the holidays and to enjoy them with contentment and ease.

You may wish to turn to page 154 for the meditation "Remember the Gift of Joy."

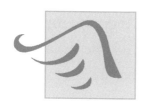

When You Are Overwhelmed

Source of All Accomplishment, I am totally overwhelmed. My task list was long before my diagnosis. Now with more medical appointments and less energy, I feel as if I am running in place. When new items appear on my agenda, when I am already not making headway, I become enormously frustrated. Sometimes my mind races forward, to calculate how to catch up, and backward, to figure out how to do things more efficiently. These frantic mental gymnastics tire me even more and add to my discouragement. Sometimes I long to ignore my responsibilities. I want to lie down and go to sleep; but I know when I awake, I will have a new rush of old concerns.

For many years, You directed me to use my talents to manage my life. You inspired me to accomplish what mattered the most for my family and work. In my time of robust health, You blessed me with efficiency and energy, freeing me to use my gifts to serve You and my loved ones.

Please slow me down, Lord. Quiet the chatter in my mind with words of comfort and wisdom. Remind me that the tortoise, not the rabbit, won the race because of a slow and steady pace. Remove the word *rush* from my vocabulary and replace it with *relax*. In Your infinite grace, grant me the vision to focus on things that truly matter: faith, family, friends, and health. Please share with me Your loving perspective and blessed peace.

You may wish to turn to page 149 for the meditation "Seeking Peace of Mind and Heart."

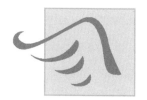

When You Are Medically Fine but Still Worried

Lord of Perfect Serenity, bless me with peace of mind—not just the freedom from a huge and immediate worry, but a deeper sense of calm in the routine activities of my life. The doctors reassure me that I am fine, and for that I am immensely grateful, but I am still uneasy. I know it takes time to recover from the physical trauma and the scars, but I did not realize the emotional impact would linger.

I longingly remember the time when I felt safe, when I did not have this cloud hovering above me. Now, I feel like there is always something in the back of my mind just waiting to slip into my consciousness and erode my security. When I forget for a while that I have had breast cancer, something reminds me of it, and my anxiety returns. I hear about a woman with a bleak prognosis. I read an article about the risks of cancer drugs. The most vivid reminders occur each day when I dress or take my medication. The most distressing reminders are the little aches or pains that plant the insidious seed that cancer lurks elsewhere yet undiagnosed.

Beloved and Peaceful God, share with me Your quiet composure. Inspire me with unfailing trust and the knowledge that events always unfold as they should, and no amount of worry will affect the outcome. Shower me with tranquility so I may feel calm about the activities of daily life. Infuse me with the optimism that expects a positive outcome. Bless me with the release of ongoing anxiety, and let me savor the comfort of Your loving presence.

You may wish to turn to page 153 for the meditation "Seeking Solid Ground."

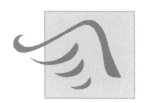

When You Are Struggling to Accept Help Graciously

Ever-present Lord, You know me as only a parent knows a child. You have seen firsthand my many attempts to be self-sufficient. You, above all, realize how challenging it is for me to allow other people do things for me—especially because I am usually the one who helps everybody else. Sometimes I wonder if I project an image of managing so well that people do not think to offer assistance.

You have blessed me with the resourcefulness to figure out solutions to my problems and the determination to forge ahead in the face of obstacles. Time and time again, I have felt Your affirming grace when I tackled a tough situation. Sometimes I dug for an answer; at other times, it burst through like a trumpet blast. Please prevent my pride in my past independence from allowing me to seek help now.

Most Precious God, I ask Your help as I struggle to relinquish my desire to be in charge of everything. Grant me the humility to stop demanding so much of myself and to embrace the generosity of others. Please let me accept help graciously and release the feeling that I am a burden. I want to surrender my independence and ask my loved ones to assist me. I know they will welcome the opportunity to minister to my needs, soothe my spirit, and serve You in the process.

You may wish to turn to page 162 for the meditation "Seeing the Big Picture."

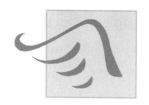

When You Are Tired of Talking About It

Dearest God, You know that I am profoundly thankful for all the people who are genuinely and lovingly concerned about my health. You know that I am especially grateful for the beloved family and friends who lift me up in prayer. I feel treasured and protected because so many people are really there for me. There lies my challenge.

I know this sounds petty and ungrateful, but, Lord, I am *so* tired of talking about breast cancer. I long to have my normal topics of conversation back, and I feel intruded upon by kind and well-meaning but endless questions. I feel like my personal space is invaded when I am faced with countless inquiries about my health. I feel like people take liberties with me without realizing it. Their questions put the cancer challenge squarely back in my mind, when I would much prefer a relaxing conversation about happy and uplifting topics. When the subject shifts to my health, I feel my energy diminish and my cheerful spirits sink.

Compassionate and Loving Lord, I know in my head that these questions are spoken with affection and concern. Maybe those who ask about my health worry that I would think they are less caring if they do not inquire. Please grant me the perspective to keep the purity of their intentions in mind and the graciousness to disguise my dismay. For those people who would understand, inspire me with the right words to gently explain that I need carefree moments when cancer is not on my mind, and sometimes I just do not want to talk about it.

You may wish to turn to page 154 for the meditation "Remember the Gift of Joy."

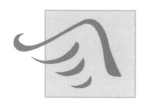

When You Are Down

Lord of Energy and Light, I am down and depleted. I lack the motivation to overcome the inertia that paralyzes me. I feel like the blues have taken up lasting residence in my life. In fact, that is the worst part of it—the inability to believe that happiness will again reside in my soul. Right now, there is nothing interesting, nothing to look forward to, no enthusiasm, no excitement. I would like to flop on the sofa, put a pillow over my head, and let someone else manage my life.

Lord, this feeling is deeply discouraging. I know it takes a great deal of energy to deal with cancer, and I should just accept the present as a time of re-gathering, renewal, and rekindling my stressed spirit. But I yearn for joy, laughter, and fun. What I feel is emptiness, boredom, and sadness.

In times too plentiful to count, You have infused my spirit with joy. You have sent precious people and delightful experiences into my life to give it meaning, purpose, and pleasure. When I am myself, I experience deep and blessed thankfulness for the glory of life. I know and trust that feeling will return.

Please remind me to be patient and to remember that healing has its own timetable and will not be rushed. Lift my spirits a little each day by reminding me to seek the things that provide pleasure and delight. Keep telling me that happiness is a curved path, and I must be willing to experience its give and take, its ebb and flow—trusting that my joy will return in time.

You may wish to turn to page 154 for the meditation "Remember the Gift of Joy."

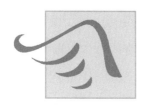

When You Are Angry

Calm and Placid Lord, I am angry. Angry that cancer happened to me. Angry that my children feel such fear. Angry about the assault on my body. Angry about the effects of the medicine. Angry with the people who steal glances at my chest. Even angrier with the ones who do not know me well yet feel perfectly free to ask me personal questions. Angry that I can no longer take for granted a long and healthy future. The ultimate anger is that cancer will always be lurking somewhere in my mind, unexpectedly making its pervasive presence known in unrelenting little ways. And I am upset that my anger brings feelings of guilt about my lack of gratitude for the loving concern and kindness shown to me.

I know that anger is normal and natural when something of this magnitude happens, but I also know it is time to move on. Lord, I need

You to help me push through this anger that drains me and ties my stomach in ugly knots. Encourage me to let go of the churning turmoil in my heart. I beseech You to guide me out of this pessimistic place, because it cannot possibly be good for my health. Sometimes it strains my relationships with those who matter most, especially Yourself.

Open my heart and my spirit to the light of Your serenity. Fill me with the strength to chase these negative thoughts from my mind so that I may turn my energy to the positive business of healing. In Your loving compassion, guide me to release this heavy load of anger so my spirit may rise to Your healing embrace.

You may wish to turn to page 157 for the meditation "Transform Resentment Into Resolve."

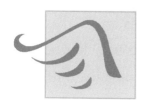

When You Need Mental Clarity

Lord of Clear Intentions, I am increasingly frustrated. Decisions that were once simple and straightforward now loom large and complicated in a cloud of uncertainty. I spend more time agonizing over small tasks, second-guessing myself, and procrastinating. Answers that were once evident now elude me. Solutions that once came quickly to mind now take detours before arriving—often too late. This decline in mental clarity makes me feel resentful and leaves me spending a lot of time struggling to catch up, keep up, and get it.

You have generously blessed me with the ability to manage my days. Sometimes it has been a scramble, but with Your help, I usually have managed to stay on top of the important things in my life. You have granted me the gifts to plan, juggle, shift gears, stay flexible, and pull it all together when the occasion demands. I am deeply grateful for these skills that I have relied on to make life run smoothly.

Giver of All Gifts, I entreat You to come to my aid as I struggle to sift through the demands and details each day brings. Illuminate my mind with Your blessed light so my vision becomes clearer and my ability to prioritize becomes stronger. Gently lift the fog that clouds my thinking and let the rays of Your brilliant love surround me. Please help me to graciously accept that my mental clarity is temporarily diminished by the stress and fatigue of my condition and to trust that it will return in time. Until then, help me to forego unnecessary tasks so I have less to overwhelm and distract me. This I ask in Your name.

You may wish to turn to page 157 for the meditation "Transform Resentment Into Resolve."

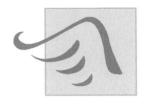

When Important Relationships Are Strained

Loving Companion, my heart is filled with sadness because my relationship with _____ _____ is suffering because of my illness. Things are strained between us, and I am painfully aware of both subtle and obvious differences. This relationship is precious to me, and I yearn for the time when our moments together were comfortable and happy. I long for the days when we shared thoughts, laughter, and hopes for the future with satisfaction and ease. I am struggling with feelings of rejection, betrayal, and distance at a time when I am vulnerable and scared.

Please know that I am grateful for the good in this relationship and the joy that it has brought to me. The happiness that I shared with _____ has enriched my life and created a treasure of memories and experiences that remain with me always.

Bless me with a mind that withholds judgment and a heart that forgives. Inspire me to understand that this dear person is having difficulty dealing with my illness and does not understand the hurt that pulling back causes me. Whether it is fear, lack of strength to see me now, or self-absorption—let me accept that each of us has weaknesses, and, in spite of them, we are still dear to You. Grant me the benevolence to focus on the positive parts of the relationship and on _____'s good qualities and to place this heartache in your compassionate hands. I am deeply comforted to know that You will never draw back from me in my hour of need.

You may wish to turn to page 142 for the meditation "Place Your Cares on the Altar of God."

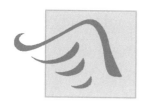

For the Strength to Take Good Care of Yourself

Lord, I realize the importance of taking good care of myself right now, but so many things get in the way and cloud my judgment. Because my energy level is low, it takes much longer to accomplish daily tasks, and then I get so far behind that I never feel caught up. Suddenly, the day is over, and I did not have the time to meditate or pray, journal, exercise, or simply to rest.

For many years, You blessed me with the vitality to manage the many priorities in my life, and I am grateful. Now I ask You to please remind me, in a firm and clear voice, that I must take care of myself. Push me out the door to take a walk, send me up the stairs to lie down, and walk me to the kitchen to take my vitamins. Create in me the unwavering belief that the things I do for myself are not options but necessities. If I will not do them for myself—or for You, because I am precious in Your eyes—then make me understand that if I exert myself to exhaustion, I will undermine my health and greatly complicate the lives of my loved ones.

Give me the grace to accept that there are times when I must put myself first and do so without guilt or apology. After I rest, I know I will better appreciate the many blessings that I still have in my life and will have renewed strength to collaborate with You and the medical team that is working hard to restore my good health.

You may wish to turn to page 162 for the meditation "Seeing the Big Picture."

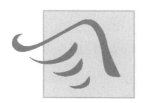

For the Return of a Sense of Humor

Lord of Laughter and Lightness, it has been too long since I enjoyed a good laugh. Before I was faced with breast cancer, I used to laugh a lot more. Now I feel so weighed down that I cannot summon my lighter side—the part of me that appreciates a funny story, laughs at a great cartoon, or savors a good comedy.

Lord, I yearn to feel the richness of Your gift of laughter again. I long to laugh until I am holding my sides and dabbing my eyes. I crave that huge post-laughter sigh, that feeling of well-being that satisfies both the body and soul. If I cannot quite scale the heights of humor, then I would truly appreciate a heart-warming chuckle or even a contagious smile. So many times in the past, You have bestowed the grace of levity upon me, and I am thankful. With Your loving help, I invite humor into my life again.

So, Dearest God, remind me to connect with the people I laugh with best, the dear friends I share funny experiences with, the delightful folks who have the ability to see the humor in everyday reality. Inspire me to seek the comedies when I watch TV or go to a movie. Motivate me to notice the cartoons in magazines and to tear out the ones I like best and post them on my refrigerator. As I gain some perspective about my own situation, grant me the insight and grace to create healing humor in my life every day, because I know it will help me to cope much better with the challenges I face.

You may wish to turn to page 151 for the meditation "Remember the Gift of Laughter."

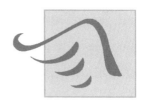

When God Seems Far Away

God, where are you? I feel disconnected and out of touch with You, and that deepens my discouragement. When I pray, I am not sure if You hear my voice. I know You have not abandoned me, but rather it is I who have wandered from You. I need to feel Your presence throughout the tedious hours of treatment, the long days of busyness or fatigue, and the lonely nights when restlessness becomes my unwelcome companion.

I yearn to feel Your loving arms around me, to know we walk each step of every day together, and we draw each breath in unison. I long for Your supportive and loving companionship to fill the lonely space within me and around me. How do I connect with You to create that deep comfort of a lifelong friend who understands my needs and accepts both my gifts and weaknesses without judgment?

Help me to know what I need to do to feel close to You again. I know that to receive, we must also give, but it is difficult to find the energy for generosity right now. I am open to Your direction, message, and guidance. I wait in silence and prayer to feel Your gentle touch. I beseech You to deepen my awareness of Your presence and ease my loneliness and fear. Speak to me, Lord, and grant me the courage to walk forward in faith.

You may wish to turn to page 159 for the meditation "Feel the Hand of God Upon Your Face."

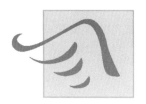

When You Feel Like Crying

Eternally Compassionate Lord, I am weeping. My heart aches with sadness and anxiety, and I desperately seek Your loving comfort. I am struggling to accept the reality of breast cancer in my life, but the uncertainty of the future—the long-term prognosis, effects of treatment, how to plan—hang like a weight on my spirit. Hearing the diagnosis shocked me, but I thought I was recovering emotionally from the news. Right now, I feel fragile, exposed, and raw. I am finding that seeds of fear, once planted, sprout roots with force and speed. Sometimes I am so frightened and discouraged that I simply cry.

Your presence in my life nourishes and consoles me. Never have I asked for the blessing of comfort that I did not sense Your arm around my shoulder. We have faced troubles together before and emerged whole, so I am confident that You will come to my aid once more. I stand before You, grateful for encouragement in the past and humbly requesting that You hear my prayer again.

Shield me from my fears and strengthen my resolve to move forward with optimism and faith. Let me experience the relief that tears bring to my bottled-up anxiety. And then, in Your everlasting compassion, I beg You to dry my tears with the holy breath of Your eternal love.

You may wish to turn to page 159 for the meditation "Feel the Hand of God Upon Your Face."

For a Friend Who Is Newly Diagnosed

Lord, I have learned that my own friend, _____ , was diagnosed with breast cancer. You know how grateful I am for the precious gift of her faithful friendship through the years. You have enriched my life immeasurably by creating the opportunity for us to meet and truly connect. The laughter and love we have shared is woven tightly into the tapestry of my life.

I beseech You to help her manage her shock and fear about her diagnosis. I remember what a loving and constant companion You were to me as I grappled with the news of my own cancer. I know that You are with us always, but sometimes our stress and anxiety obscure our vision. Please surround her with the light of Your compassion and allow her to feel Your comforting presence. Inspire her to reach for Your hand every time she awaits a lab report, sits in the waiting room, or considers a treatment.

And Loving God, please enlighten me with ideas for being a caring and supportive friend. Let me borrow from Your example of divine friendship and offer to her all the love and practical help I can.

You may wish to turn to page 170 for the meditation "Bearing a Message of God's Love."

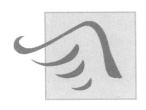

For All Women With Breast Cancer

Lord of all Creation, by virtue of my breast cancer, You have connected me with countless women who share my situation and understand my concerns as only You can. We have forged the unbreakable bond of a shared, painful experience. We stand united in our daily challenges, our ongoing anxieties, and our fervent hopes for a tomorrow that brings a cure.

The support I receive from my sister survivors enriches my life and enhances my strength. I am thankful that we stand united in a magnificent circle of caring. Those who are able to give provide comfort and inspire courage for those who need to receive. And the circle shifts to embrace new members in an ever-widening network of kindness and empathy.

Bless each one of them with strength of spirit as she journeys along this unexpected path. Grant them healing of body and mind so they may honor and serve You by providing information and encouragement to others. I ask You to be ever-present in their lives as they turn to You each day for inspiration and support. Above all, infuse them with the indomitable faith that You will be there for them always and in all ways.

You may wish to turn to page 170 for the meditation "Bearing a Message of God's Love."

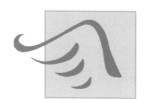

For the Wisdom to Find the Good in This Experience

Dearest Lord, I know that painful experiences can be blessings in disguise, but I am struggling with this idea right now. I am having great difficulty understanding how my fear and uncertainty—and that of my family—will lead to a greater good. I am trying valiantly to deal with the constant exposing and touching of my body by strangers by remembering that their intent is to help and heal me. I am absorbing the shock to my security and wondering what insights will eventually emerge.

Am I to be an example of courage for others? Will this experience teach me patience? Can I make the time to nurture myself without hearing nagging little whispers that I should be busy? Will I finally slow down? Can I see my priorities with greater clarity? Will I someday be a source of comfort for other women?

In the midst of my struggle, I offer my gratitude for the opportunity to grow in wisdom and in depth. I trust that the emotional pain will bring me perspective.

Help me to accept that every problem comes with a gift in its hands. Guide me to believe that there is a larger purpose behind these weeks and months of treatment. Give me the gift of discernment that I may see with clear eyes how I can eventually transform this experience into something positive. Only by doing this will I be able to stop resisting the way cancer has irrevocably changed my life. Inspire me to pause, and peer closely at my life with the intent to shed thoughts and behaviors that are no longer useful. Above all, enable me to lovingly support other women who struggle with breast cancer.

You may wish to turn to page 163 for the meditation "Open Your Heart to Wisdom."

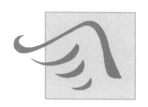

Thanksgiving for Supportive Family*

For Supportive Spouse:

Bountiful Lord, I stand before You in profound gratitude for the extraordinary blessing of my loving and supportive spouse. He has walked beside me from the first step of this unexpected challenge—always present, never faltering. He encouraged me when fatigue and frustration filled me, consoled me when sadness filled my spirit, and inspired me with his steadfast devotion. I feel humbled at the magnitude of such a precious gift.

Although I never would have chosen to take this journey, his presence at my side has strengthened me to continue my treatment with calm resolve. His optimism about the future protected me from my own sadness. His quiet courage and shining faith in Your presence nourishes my spirit and fills me with admiration. My heart overflows with thanksgiving that You have brought a person of such goodness and generosity into my life.

Please recognize him as Your devoted servant and shower him with abundant blessings.

For Supportive Children:

Eternal and Compassionate Parent, you know how pleased You are when we, Your children, live our lives as reflections of Your brilliant Light. I am filled with gratitude for the caring and courageous spirit shown by my children during my treatment. Their encouragement and prayers inspired me to stand tall when confronting fear and to be diligent about my treatment in the face of fatigue.

Bless them for their attention and helpfulness when I needed their care. Reward them for their abundant caring by drawing into their lives people like themselves who love without restraint and serve without hesitation. Fill their lives with Your love and keep them close to You always. As Your loving child, I speak this heartfelt plea.

You may wish to turn to page 155 for the meditation "Sing a Song of Thanksgiving."

You may adapt these prayers to include partner, siblings, other relatives, and any people with whom you share "family" relationships.

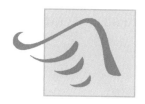

Thanksgiving for Supportive Friends

Lord of Companionship and Comfort, You have blessed me with the priceless gift of supportive friends. They have helped immensely to make this journey of breast cancer care more bearable and less lonely. My dear friends have accompanied me to appointments, provided healthy and comforting meals, and helped me with practical tasks. They have soothed my spirit, listened to my concerns with undying patience and love, and encouraged me to go deep inside myself and find my own strength. Most of all, they have lifted me up in prayer that You would shine Your healing light upon me and give me the perseverance to endure whatever treatments I choose.

Lord, in your infinite wisdom, You give us the capacity to form loving and lasting friendships that enhance our joy and diminish the toll our trials take on our spirits. Thank you for sending loyal and loving friends who provide practical and emotional support and who surround me with tender care. Please shower them with abundant blessings, especially the support of good friends in their own lives. Inspire me to demonstrate by my own actions that the love of friendship is reciprocal and enduring.

For my friends' unwavering and ever-present support and love, for their constant kindness, prayers, and the richness they bring into my life, in both good times and bad, I offer humble and heartfelt thanks.

You may wish to turn to page 155 for the meditation "Sing a Song of Thanksgiving."

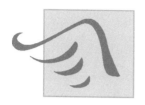

Thanksgiving for Faithful Pets

Master of All Creation, Your abundant world teems with splendid creatures that bring joy and satisfaction into our lives. Each animal represents a unique and wondrous perfection with its own personality, nature, and habits. From the great to the small, the fierce to the timid, the cuddly to the aloof, the scope of Your kingdom fills my soul with awe at the grandeur of Your creation. Your magnificence reveals itself in the vast spectrum of glorious creatures that fill the land, air, and sea.

I am especially blessed to have _____ (name of pet) in my life right now when my security has been shaken, and fears about the future fly unbidden into my mind. When I feel anxious, his unconditional love and loyalty lifts my spirits and distracts me from my concerns. How reinforcing to look into his trusting and eager eyes. Thank you for bringing this source of deep affection and total acceptance into my life.

As I beseech Your blessing for my own health and well-being, I also ask You to shine endless grace on my faithful and beloved companion, who has brought me enormous consolation and quiet joy during this challenging time.

You may wish to turn to page 166 for the meditation "Glorify All of God's Creatures."

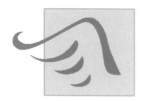

Thanksgiving for Everyday Joys

Lord of Abundance, in the midst of anxiety and fatigue, I search for—and find—a multitude of little miracles in the daily routine of my life. Each one nourishes my soul and bolsters me to stay the course. The blessed brilliance of sunshine on my face as I wait for a traffic light to change. The little children who shed coats on the first warm day of spring. The purple intensity of feisty crocuses that flaunt the end of winter. The lingering fragrance of herbal shampoo in my daughter's hair as she brushes my cheek in a "gotta go" good-bye. The expectant "I-live-for-this-moment" face of a black Labrador awaiting a chunk of cheddar. The rush of loving pleasure at a thinking-of-you card from a treasured friend.

Your bountiful blessings give me respite from anxiety and remind me that even as I confront breast cancer, Your world still teems with infinite treasure. I need only to slow down, notice, and admire. Then I feel my spirit expand with the gratitude of one who is learning to see with new eyes.

Let me continue to inhale with awe at a flaming orange sunset. May the luxury of rose petals always gladden my fingertips. Bless me with happy contentment at that place where favorite old melodies and memories meet. Sustain the intensity of my joy at hearing the surf crash upon the shore. Deepen my delight in the simple pleasure of warm apple pie and cold vanilla ice cream. Most Generous God, I yearn to fix in my mind and heart the gratitude I feel at this moment. I ask that in Your boundless generosity, You show me the way.

You may wish to turn to page 155 for the meditation "Sing a Song of Thanksgiving."

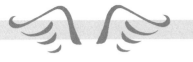

Introduction to Meditations

Each meditation can stand alone, or it can follow a specific prayer. Whatever feels right to you *is* right. The only important thing is that this volume will bring to you a measure of companionship, serenity, and hope, however you choose to use it.

You may wish to read through the meditation once before you actually begin it. That way you will be focused on the experience and not on the directions. And always, before you begin, take three slow and relaxed breaths to ease the tensions of the day and open your mind and heart to healing.

After you have completed a meditation several times and are familiar with it, you may wish to close your eyes during the process. If you are seated during the meditation, you may wish to let your hands rest gently in your lap, with palms upward to receive the flow of God's grace. If you are lying down, choose whatever posture promotes deep relaxation.

Part Six:
Meditations to
Calm Your Spirit

"I have discovered the secret of the
sea in meditation upon a dewdrop."
—*Kahlil Gibran*

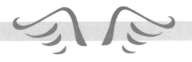

Place Your Cares on the Altar of God

Take three slow and deep breaths to release the tensions of the day.

Imagine a beautiful altar made of the finest marble. It is covered with an ivory cloth that is finely embroidered with the religious symbols of your faith. The altar is surrounded by golden light that resembles a fine mist. The sun shines through and illuminates the altar so that it appears to glow softly. You feel the presence of God as you look at the altar, and you wish to approach it. You hear a gentle voice inviting you to come closer and leave your burdens there.

Visualize yourself placing your fears into a box. Wrap it lovingly, as if it were an exquisite gift, because your burdens and everything about you are precious to God. Approach the altar, and climb the seven steps that represent all the days of the week when you worry. Tell the Lord that your mind and heart are weary, and that you wish to be relieved of your concerns for a time. Place your box on the altar, and humbly request that the Lord take care of your problems while you rest and restore yourself. Bow and walk down the steps, feeling the relief of knowing that you are never alone at any time, especially when your heart is heavy.

Take three more slow and deep breaths before returning to your tasks or going to sleep. If you feel burdened with worry again during the day or wake during the night, know that your cares are out of your hands for now, safe on the altar of God.

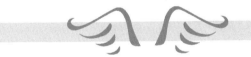

Direct Treatments to Their Target

Take three slow and deep breaths to release the tensions of the day.

Imagine (or in reality) you are waiting for a chemotherapy or radiation treatment. Your session is about to begin, and the nurse or technician is making the final adjustments while talking to you in a calm and reassuring way. You feel optimistic about the results of the procedure. Your intent is to cooperate fully in mind, body, and spirit to maximize the positive effects. You mentally scan your body, and with a small brush, whisk away any emotional debris—anxiety, resistance, anger—that could stand in the way of the treatment.

Now visualize the chemotherapy agent or radiation beam traveling through your body, seeking and easily finding its targeted cells. There are no barriers between unwanted cells and the treatment, so the invaders are quickly identified and their energy destroyed. Your healthy cells are happy with more room to thrive. The remnants of the unwelcome visitors are flushed from your body, and the healing process continues as you surrender to the blessing of the treatment.

Continue your slow and deep breathing for as long as you wish as you see the healing agents travel to their target.

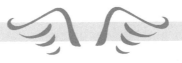

Create a Veil of Love for Your Head

Take three slow and deep breaths to release the tensions of the day.

Imagine that you are seated in the middle of a circle of the people who are most important to you—beloved family members, dear and cherished friends, loved ones who have gone on to the next life. Slowly look around the circle and rest your gaze briefly on each of their faces. Observe the deep caring and kindness in their eyes. Each one of them is here to lift up your spirits with their devotion and loyalty. Breathe deeply and feel the abundant blessing of the love that surrounds you.

Visualize each person coming forward and offering you soft strands of a beautiful cloth in many shades of a color that is one of your favorites. The hues range from delicately soft to vibrantly bold. Choose in your mind the person with whom you feel the strongest heart connection, and beckon that person to come forward to you. Hand her the strands of cloth and watch her weave them into a radiant veil of love for your head. Bow slightly, and allow her to drape it gently while you experience the collective love of those you cherish. Let your heart and your eyes speak your gratitude to your circle.

Continue your slow and deep breathing for as long as you wish. You may rest your hands very lightly on your head to "feel" your veil.

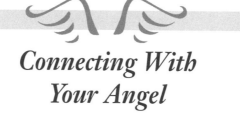

Connecting With Your Angel

Take three slow and deep breaths to release the tensions of the day.

Visualize a radiant angel standing behind you and enveloping your shoulders with luminous wings. You feel calmed and stabilized by the presence of this heavenly guardian, and you close your eyes for a minute to appreciate the sense of peace that surrounds you. You then wish to see your angel's face, and you turn slowly to look at her.

You gaze at a face that reflects profound compassion for you. Feel the warmth and hear the calm, even breathing of this glorious being who walks with you always. Speak to her of your worries, and sense the strength of her wings as a shield against your deepest anxieties. Her constant and loving presence is a protective shawl that surrounds you with love and support. Tell her that you are releasing your fears to the light of her protection.

Continue your slow and deep breathing for as long as you wish while you feel your angel's touch on your shoulders.

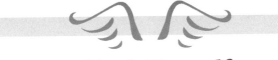

Cloak Yourself With Courage

Take three slow and deep breaths to release the tensions of the day.

Imagine that many bolts of luxurious cloth surround you. There are gently draping silks in soft and vibrant hues, rich and colorful tweeds, regal satins, and plush velvets. You wish to choose a length of special fabric to wrap around you like a flowing cape. Gently touch the weave of each, and let your eyes respond to the colors and your fingers to the textures. Trust yourself to make the ideal selection that will inspire you to feel strong and courageous.

Visualize yourself bringing the fabric around to cover your back, letting the ends drape down in front of you. Now wrap them closely around your shoulders and say to yourself, "I am clothed in the courage of my Creator." Know that your cloak of courage is a protective garment you can don at any time to remind you that the Lord will always shield you and provide you with inner strength.

Continue your slow and deep breathing for as long as you wish as you feel the cloth on your shoulders.

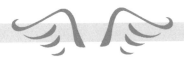

Seeking Peace of Mind and Heart

Take three slow and deep breaths to release the tensions of the day.

Imagine that you are sitting in a room that is furnished with a white sofa and chairs of simple fabric. A loosely woven white area rug covers a brilliant golden oak floor. The afternoon sun shines through sheer curtains that billow in a gentle breeze. On the coffee table, there is a leather-bound book with gilt-edged pages containing the most important truths of your faith. The simplicity and silence of the room make it feel both serene and spiritual.

Visualize the Lord slowly entering the room, surrounded by a soft light that resembles a morning mist. As the Lord draws nearer to you, the light becomes golden. The Divine Master takes a chair and reads a passage from the book that seems intended just for you: "Be still, my soul, and open thyself to peace. Be still, my soul, and open thyself to peace," again and again. The Lord's voice is gentle and reassuring as He invites you to repeat this message in your mind until it is written on your heart. "Be still, my soul, and open thyself to peace."

Continue your slow and deep breathing for as long as you wish. You may want to repeat "Be still, my soul, and open thyself to peace" each time you exhale.

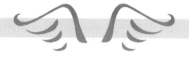

Wrap Your Children in a Quilt of God's Love

Take three slow and deep breaths to release the tensions of the day.

Imagine yourself sorting through a box of special garments that your children have worn: a holiday outfit, a costume from a school play, an infant sleeper, a graduation gown. You touch each item tenderly to your cheek and reminisce about the occasion of its wearing. The cherished memories lift up your spirits and fill your heart with love for your children. You yearn to protect them from all harm and fear.

Visualize a remarkable quilt containing small patches of the garments you just touched with such tenderness. The beautiful and unique pattern depicts hearts within hearts, the outer ones the glorious sky blue of God's creation, the inner ones created from the fabrics of your children's history. In your mind, pick up the quilt and wrap it tenderly around your children, touching each one on the cheek and asking for God's protection. Know that the love of the Lord surrounds your children now and always.

Continue your slow and deep breathing for as long as you wish as you feel the protective presence of God's love.

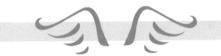

Remember the Gift of Laughter

Take three slow and deep breaths to release the tensions of the day.

Imagine yourself getting together with the people you laugh with the most. They are the ones who can tell the story of an ordinary day through the extraordinary eyes of humor. They make mundane events delightfully mirthful. If you ever laughed until you cried, it was with them. If you ever felt so weak from laughing that you had to sit down, it was on their chairs. Feel the bubbling energy of their presence.

Visualize each one handing you a package— no fancy wrappings, just plain paper and colorful string. You open each one to find a memory of shared laughter, sometimes rippling with warmth, sometimes howling with hilarity. Line them up on a low table and sit down to examine them. Select one of your favorites and re-experience it in vivid detail. Laugh as you recollect it either to yourself or out loud, and trust that when this challenge is over, laughter will again emerge vibrant and strong.

Continue your slow and deep breathing for as long as you wish, and imagine the Lord sharing your laughter.

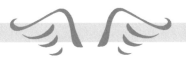

Seeking Solid Ground

Take three slow and deep breaths to release the tensions of the day.

Imagine that you are a tall and sturdy oak tree, part of an ancient and towering grove. See your body as a solid trunk. You know that you have survived many fierce winds and raging storms. Your tough network of roots has projected downward and outward with the passage of time. After the stress of every life storm, you have become more firmly planted.

Visualize that your feet are growing roots deep into the earth, connecting with nature's basic instinct to grow and thrive. These tenacious roots anchor you firmly to the ground. They are dependable and strong, and you can rely on them to keep you standing. Feel a surge of energy from the bottom of your feet pushing your roots deeper to create an even more secure place to stand. Breathe deeply and know that you are safe and firmly grounded in God's love.

Continue your deep and slow breathing for as long as you wish. You may want to do this meditation in a standing position to create more of a "rooted" feeling.

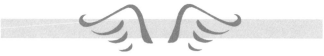

Remember the Gift of Joy

Take three slow and deep breaths to release the tensions of the day.

Let your mind wander and recall several of your happiest moments: a memorable occasion with loved ones; the miracle of a child's birth; a meaningful accomplishment; an unexpected surprise; a loving comment that made you feel valued. Each one of these experiences is a rare and precious coin that adds value to your life. Your collection of happy memories has made you wealthy beyond measure. Each one was a deposit in your personal account of life joy. Each one was a blessing from a Loving Creator.

Visualize yourself entering a bank that is bright with natural light and decorated with many lush green plants. You approach the manager who greets you with a smile and offers to help. Explain that you wish to borrow from your account to experience joy until your sadness and stress diminish. Examine each precious deposit in minute detail. Fill your heart and nourish your spirit with remembered joy. Trust that life will bring many more uplifting and positive experiences to enlarge your account and enrich your life.

Continue your deep and slow breathing for as long as you wish as you think about your experiences of joy.

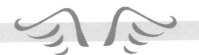

Sing a Song of Thanksgiving

Take three slow and deep breaths to release the tensions of the day.

Imagine that you have been blessed with a lovely singing voice, worthy of performance. The melodies that you sing resonate with bright and pure tones. Because you sing from the heart, you connect deeply with all who hear your voice. You feel humble and grateful to use this gift to praise God and serve others.

Visualize yourself standing on a stage dressed in a deep blue choir robe. A huge chorus of magnificent angels surrounds you. As if from some unseen cue, they begin to sing, each note filled with vitality and boundless joy. The lyrics are profoundly simple and moving: "My soul overflows with gratitude for blessings great and small." You join your voice with theirs, delighted that you blend in perfectly. You feel the words in the very fiber of your being. "My soul overflows with gratitude for blessings great and small." The choir of angels begins to sing more softly until your radiant voice is the only sound. You know that your gratitude will travel straight to the heart of God.

Continue your deep and slow breathing for as long as you wish as you hear in your mind the beautiful simplicity of your song.

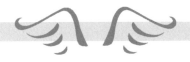

Transform Resentment
Into Resolve

Take three slow and deep breaths to release the tensions of the day.

Imagine that each flash of anger you experience is a rectangular gray stone in a wall of resentment that separates you from the place you desire. The barricade rises too high for you to see over, but is low enough for you to reach up and touch the top row. As you visually scan the stones, you notice lightly etched markings that identify the source of each resentment: cancer, fatigue, rude treatment at an appointment, lack of support from a loved one, whatever happened that diminished your vitality, optimism, and joy.

Visualize yourself removing a stone from the top row. Read what it says and pick up a file and gently erase the etching of your anger. Continue to do this with each stone, placing it on the ground in a series of risers that form a sturdy staircase. When the wall is halfway down, the steps will raise high enough to climb over the wall. With half of the burden of anger released, the remainder will lose its hold over you. Cross over toward peace by treading on the remnants of resentment.

Continue your slow and deep breathing for as long as you wish as you visualize yourself stepping over anger into peace.

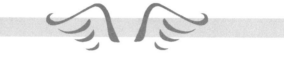

Activate Your Healing Energy

Take three slow and deep breaths to release the tensions of the day.

Imagine yourself sitting at the summit of a low mountain that stands apart from the rest of the range. The sun has just descended below the horizon, leaving a twilight sky of deep rose with streaks of purple. Your attention is captured by the uncommon hues of the sunset, and you experience a sense of awe at the wonders of creation. You breathe deeply and savor the quiet glory of day's end.

Visualize yourself stretching your arms to the sky. Your hands are wide open with palms facing up. Focus your intent on asking the Lord to infuse you with healing energy. Breathe deeply and invite the energy to enter your body through your outstretched hands. Imagine your palms feeling slightly warm as the flow of the Lord's healing power begins to travel through your body. See the energy as a river of white light moving through your body and gathering strength as it connects with your own immune system.

Continue your slow and deep breathing for as long as you wish as you express gratitude for your healing partnership with the Divine Physician.

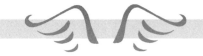

Feel the Hand of God Upon Your Face

Take three slow and deep breaths to release the tensions of the day.

Imagine yourself entering a small stone building housing a place of worship that is sacred to your faith. You feel drawn slowly down the center aisle toward an altar by a gentle force that is outside of you. There is a magnetic quality about the altar that beckons but does not insist. You relax and surrender to the pull and find yourself directly in front of the altar with your head bowed in reverence. You hear soft music that you recognize as a hymn from your childhood. You sense that something of great importance is about to happen, and you become peacefully alert.

Raise your head to see the Lord clothed in a simple white robe standing behind the altar and looking at you with warm recognition. Nothing else exists at this moment except the loving bond of your eyes. Watch Him walk slowly around the altar toward you and extend a warm hand to touch your cheek in a gesture of love so profound that it reaches the depth of your soul. You close your eyes to capture the moment as your heart overflows with gratitude. Breathe deeply and know that you can call forth the memory by touching your own hand on your face and focusing on God's abiding love.

Continue your slow and deep breathing for as long as you wish as you rest one hand gently on your face.

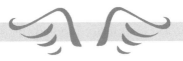

Call Forth Light in the Midst of Darkness

Take three slow and deep breaths to release the tensions of the day.

Picture yourself walking with God along a lovely and secluded beach. The roar of the surf fills your ears with its thunderous power. The sun sets over the water as the two of you stop to admire the evening sky painted with blazing streaks of orange. The sun slips below the horizon, and night falls quickly. Darkness completely envelops you, and although you can no longer see the Lord, you experience a sense of safety and warmth.

You feel God reach for your hand, urging you gently to look in the other direction, away from the water. Day breaks suddenly over the land with dazzling glory. The sun rises overhead and chases away the lingering shadows as you marvel at the miracle of the fleeting darkness. You and the Lord are bathed in splendid sunlight. You close your eyes and raise your face to the sun as God lovingly whispers in your ear, "My dearest child, I will surround you with my light any time you desire. You need simply to ask."

Continue slow and deep breathing, and hold this image for as long as you wish.

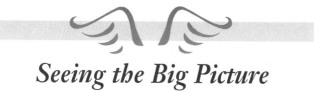

Seeing the Big Picture

Take three slow and deep breaths to release the tensions of the day.

Imagine that you are standing in front of a large mirror that is draped with a soft white cloth. A small slice of the mirror is visible on the left side, allowing you to see just your face. You see concern and fatigue, as well as hope and determination, in your eyes. You study your image carefully, searching for signs that your vitality and energy will return. Your face reflects the burden you carry, but, unmistakably, a new strength is evident.

Visualize yourself very slowly removing the cloth from the mirror. Standing behind you, but reflected in front of you, are all the loved ones who pray for and support you. They stood watch with you through this challenge so far and will continue going forward with you. Look carefully in the mirror again to see images of dear ones who have gone to the next life. They know your concerns and bring unconditional love and support. Gaze in the mirror a final time to see the Lord at your side, quietly putting an arm around your shoulder to accompany you through this challenging chapter of your life.

Continue your slow and deep breathing as you gaze into the mirror for as long as you wish.

Open Your Heart to Wisdom

Take three slow and deep breaths to release the tensions of the day.

Imagine that you have been told that a very wise and holy woman lives at the edge of an untouched section of forest not far from your home.

Trusted friends assure you that she welcomes visitors who seek to hear the voice of their own inner wisdom. You wish to visit with her and share the concerns that cast a long shadow on your happiness. You know that she accepts no payment, so you take her a gift—a small, covered crystal container in the shape of a heart.

Visualize yourself walking up the sun-dappled path to her modest cottage. She opens the door and greets you warmly and asks the Lord to bless you as you enter her home. You give her the crystal heart, which she graciously accepts and removes the lid from. She invites you to a comfortable sitting area and you share the concerns of your heart while her kind eyes never leave your face. When you have finished speaking, you realize that you already know your answers. The wise woman places the container in your hands as you leave, but she keeps the lid. She tells you to reflect quietly and always keep your heart open when you seek wisdom.

Continue your slow and deep breathing for as long as you wish, with your right hand placed gently over your heart.

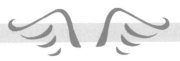

Search for Sun in Gray Skies

Take three slow and deep breaths to release the tensions of the day.

Imagine that you have made plans for a day of relaxation at an ocean or lake beach. The sun is shining when you arrive, but as morning turns into afternoon, the sky becomes overcast, turning the color of an old aluminum baking pan. You can discern a faint outline of the sun behind the cloud cover, but it seems unable to gather the intensity to break through.

Visualize yourself walking to the water's edge and staring directly at the precise spot in the sky where the sun hides. Speak to the sun in your mind and invite it to resume shining its healing rays directly on the earth. Put your arms together and extend them in front of you toward the sun. Now slowly separate them as if gently parting the curtain of clouds that obscures the light you seek. Turn your face to the heavens, close your eyes, and feel the warmth envelop you.

Continue your slow and deep breathing as long as you wish while you hold in your mind an image of the healing sun.

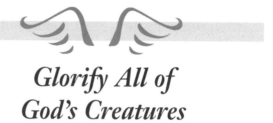

Glorify All of God's Creatures

Take three slow and deep breaths to release the tensions of the day.

Imagine that you were present to witness the creation of the world. You watched silently as the Divine Creator breathed life into the cosmos and started the events culminating in the creation of all creatures. The dazzling array of great and small, wild and tame, furry and smooth filled your heart with awe and joy. You have recalled the splendor many times and re-create in your mind the sublime wonder of that day.

Visualize yourself looking out over a teeming sea of life. You gaze across a vast expanse and see every creature in its uniqueness and glory. You are enthralled to witness this immense array of animals, and you praise God for the beauty and variety of it all. Most of the creatures move quietly away, while a few that touch your heart most come forward and gently nuzzle your hand. You stand very still to savor the experience and feel your spirit expand with wondrous delight.

Continue your slow and deep breathing for as long as you wish while you think in vivid detail about the animals you love most dearly.

Surround Caregivers With Grace

Take three slow and deep breaths to release the tensions of the day.

Visualize yourself in an attractive meeting room in the hospital where you have been receiving treatment. The room is decorated with uplifting paintings of loving families and friends and majestic nature scenes. The forest green furnishings create an inviting atmosphere. All of the medical caregivers—doctors, nurses, and technicians—who helped to restore your health are assembled in a single row of seats facing you. The doors at the back of the room are open.

In a clear, vibrant voice, you call out the name of each person, beckoning them to the front of the room. As each steps forward, other patients and their families enter through the rear doors and walk to the front of the room. They form a circle around the care providers. You join the circle, and all clasp hands and ask the Lord to bless these honored people with continued compassion and the grace to regard their work as a healing ministry. The group expresses deep gratitude for care received, and after each person is mentioned and blessed, all return quietly to continue their work.

Continue your slow and deep breathing while you hold the image of those who care for you being surrounded by God's grace.

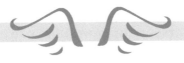

Staying on Course

Take three slow and deep breaths to release the tensions of the day.

Visualize yourself leaving your home for a drive to a lovely cottage on a lake several hours away. A friend has offered you the use of the property for a few days. Because it is one of your favorite places, you savor the thought of the trip. You leave with plenty of time to arrive before dark. The beginning of the journey is pleasant and you enjoy the crisp and vibrant green of the spring day.

An hour into the journey you become ensnarled in heavy traffic, inching along to discover a closed lane. Eventually, you remember a secondary road and turn off, but miles later, find yourself facing a sign announcing a closed bridge. Momentarily discouraged, thoughts of returning home enter your mind, but the lure of the lake is strong. You return to the highway to discover traffic moving faster now, and you stay on course, pulling into the driveway much later than expected. You are greeted by a sunset so spectacular you stop and stare in awe. Moved by the beauty, you enter the cottage to find a welcoming note from your dear friend. You light the fire and sit down to read the note again, nourished by nature and friendship.

Continue your slow and deep breathing for as long as you wish while you hold the image of yourself sitting by the fire, warmed and happy that you persevered.

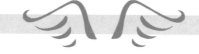

Bearing a Message of God's Love

Take three slow and deep breaths to release the tensions of the day.

Visualize yourself seated in a quiet house of worship that touches your soul with its beauty and serenity. The sun's rays filter through many tall windows and surround the altar with soft light. You feel moved to approach the altar, where you find a small decorative silver tray on which a cream-colored linen envelope rests. You notice, to your surprise, that your name is on the envelope.

You carefully lift the envelope flap, remove a sheet of paper, and begin to read. "Beloved Daughter, I know you feel great compassion for all women with breast cancer, especially those who reside in fear. Reassure them with words or with the voice of your heart that I am ever present with each one of them. Encourage them to come to me for protection from anxiety and for the comfort of my enduring love." You hold the message to your heart and whisper your gratitude and willingness to serve as a humble messenger.

Continue your slow and deep breathing as you picture yourself conveying the Lord's message to other women with breast cancer. For some, you may use words; for others, the intent of your heart delivers the message.

Part Seven:
Prayer Resources to Ensure That You Are Never Alone

"More things are wrought by prayer than the world dreams of."
— *Alfred, Lord Tennyson*

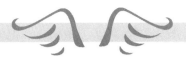

Guidelines for Prayer Resources

It is important to preface the following resources with some thoughts on the nature and effectiveness of prayer. When people pray for your intentions, they are asking the Lord to provide you with a benefit. For women undergoing treatment for breast cancer, certainly the most frequent petition will be for the restoration of health. Our prayers and those of our loved ones will most likely focus on requests for successful surgery, remission, relief from side effects of treatment, and survival.

Please bear in mind that participation in prayer ministries does not guarantee the results that we desire.

How and why some prayers appear to be "answered" and some not remains a mystery. Even though we may have many people—family, friends, and strangers—praying on our behalf, this does not necessarily translate into an affirmative answer to our prayers. Although it is certainly beneficial to remain optimistic and hopeful about our petitions, we also need to know that not every request will come to pass.

However, many prayers will be answered in the way we desire. Some may experience a cure, but most will experience the healing power of prayer in the form of comfort and consolation, relief from anxiety, and reassurance of the presence of a loving and personal God who is always with us.

Please read the following guidelines before contacting any of the prayer resources.

1. The information that follows was correct at the time of publication, but please be aware that Web addresses occasionally change or become unavailable. If you are unable to access a particular group, you can try entering the name of the organization as a keyword, or simply move on to another organization.

2. Some of these organizations request information from you (e.g., name, e-mail address). Others request first name only. Still others permit you to remain anonymous

if you wish. You will need to decide how much information you wish to submit.

3. There is no fee for making a prayer request, and my experience has been that I do not receive solicitations for donations even from those organizations where I provided my name. My donations to some of them have been at my initiative. However, if you choose to make a contribution, no doubt it will be gratefully received, as some of these groups rely on gifts to meet their operating expenses. But I stress that this is entirely up to you.

4. Inclusion on this list is not an endorsement of the organization. No formal review of these organizations was conducted. You may wish to visit their Web sites to determine if their missions correlate with your own religious beliefs.

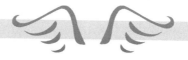

Prayer Resources

The resources that follow are only a few of many organizations that respond to prayer requests. These are all national organizations that accept petitions from anyone desiring prayer. Many of these organizations are nondenominational, and it is not necessary that you be a member of the organization or the same religious faith to request intercessory prayer.

You can locate thousands of more intercessory prayer groups on the Internet by entering the keywords "prayer ministries." You may wish to explore the resources in your geographical area and contact your local parish or congregation and request prayers for your intentions. Also, many cities have a Council of Churches that may be able to help you locate a prayer ministry that would be suitable for your beliefs.

World Network of Prayer
www.wnop.org

Visit the site and click on "Submit a Request" and enter your petition, or you may e-mail their office at pray@wnop.org. The World Network of Prayer is operated by the United Pentecostal Church International. In addition to accepting and distributing prayer requests, they observe the National Day of Prayer and the World Day of Prayer.

Silent Unity
www.unityworldhq.org

Silent Unity is a worldwide prayer ministry that has been in continuous ministry with people of all faiths for more than 100 years. Someone is always praying in the chapel, 24 hours a day, 365 days a year. You may visit their Web site and enter a prayer request that will be enfolded in continuous prayer for 30 days. The site is affiliated with the Unity School of Christianity that is based on the teachings of Jesus and the healing power of prayer.

American Catholic
www.Americancatholic.org

Visit their Web site and click on "Prayer Intentions." Type your intention in the box provided. Your prayers will be forwarded to an editor for posting on the prayer intentions board. They also will be presented on the following Tuesday morning among the prayers at the National Shrine of St. Anthony in Cincinnati, Ohio. You may re-enter your petition weekly if you desire.

Prayer Ministries International
www.pray4you.com

Prayer Ministries International is a non-profit ministry aspiring to encourage a Christ-centered prayer relationship between those who desire prayer and those who welcome the opportunity to pray on their behalf. Your request can be submitted anonymously or with identifying information. Your request is transmitted to the prayer coordinator who forwards it to "prayer partners." They will pray for your request each day for one week, after which you may submit it again.

Self-Realization Fellowship Prayer Council
www.yogananda-srf.org

Self-Realization Fellowship Prayer Council is a worldwide religious organization dedicated to carrying on the spiritual and humanitarian work of Paramahansa Yogananda, a revered spiritual leader and native of India. Each morning and evening, the prayer council prays for the physical, mental, and spiritual healing of all whose names have been given to them. Requests remain with the prayer council for three months.

Sisters of St. Francis of Perpetual Adoration
www.ssfpa.org

Enter their Web site and click on "Prayer Requests." You may enter your e-mail address or remain anonymous. They will bring your intentions before the Lord in their Perpetual Adoration chapel during their unceasing hours of prayer where at least two of the sisters are in prayer throughout the day and night. The Sisters of St. Francis of Perpetual Adoration are a Catholic order of nuns who strive to combine the contemplative life of prayer with the active life of perpetual adoration and works of mercy.

Guideposts
www.guideposts.org

Enter their Web site and click on "Request Prayer." You may send a private prayer request that will be viewed only by staff or a volunteer committed to pray specifically for your needs. Or, you may post a public prayer request on their Web site, and your request will be prayed for by a prayer volunteer and any Web visitors wishing to pray online. You are requested to use your first name only to protect your privacy and the privacy of others.